Better Sleep
for your
Baby & Child

Better Sleep
for your
Baby & Child

A Parent's Step-by-Step Guide to Healthy Sleep Habits

Dr. Shelly K. Weiss, MD, FRCPC
with
Mark Feldman, MD, FRCPC
James MacFarlane BSc, MSc, PhD
Ian B. MacLusky, MBBS, FRCPC
Golda Milo-Manson, MHSc, MD, FRCPC
Eileen P. Sloan, MD, PhD, FRCPC
Robyn Stremler, RN, PhD

The Hospital for Sick Children

Robert
ROSE

To my daughters, Abby and Jenna, my first and best teachers about sleep in children.

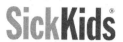

Disclaimer

This book is a general guide only and should never be a substitute for the skill, knowledge, and experience of a qualified medical professional dealing with the facts, circumstances, and symptoms of a particular case.

The nutritional, medical, and health information presented in this book is based on the research, training, and professional experience of the authors, and is true and complete to the best of their knowledge. However, this book is intended only as an informative guide for those wishing to know more about health, nutrition, and medicine; it is not intended to replace or countermand the advice given by the reader's personal physician. Because each person and situation is unique, the authors and the publisher urge the reader to check with a qualified health-care professional before using any procedure where there is a question as to its appropriateness. A physician should be consulted before beginning any exercise program. The authors and the publisher are not responsible for any adverse effects or consequences resulting from the use of the information in this book. It is the responsibility of the reader to consult a physician or other qualified health-care professional regarding his or her personal care.

Library and Archives Canada Cataloguing in Publication

Weiss, Shelly K
      Better sleep for your baby & child: a parent's step-by-step guide to healthy sleep habits / Shelly K. Weiss.

Includes index.
ISBN-13: 978-0-7788-0149-8
ISBN-10: 0-7788-0149-7

1. Children — Sleep. 2. Sleep disorders in children — Prevention. 3. Child rearing. I. Title.

RJ506.S55W43 2006   649'.4   C2006-902634-3

Edited by Bob Hilderley, Senior Editor, Health.
Copyedited by Fina Scroppo.
Index by Gillian Watts.
Design and page composition by PageWave Graphics Inc.
Cover image: Rommel/Masterfile

The publisher acknowledges the financial support of the Government of Canada through the Book Publishing Industry Development Program.

Published by Robert Rose Inc.
120 Eglinton Ave. E., Suite 800, Toronto, Ontario Canada M4P 1E2
Tel: (416) 322-6552 Fax: (416) 322-6936

Printed and bound in Canada.

1 2 3 4 5 6 7 8 9 CPL 14 13 12 11 10 09 08 07 06

Contents

Contributors. 6
Introduction. 7

Part 1: Healthy Sleep
1. Sleep Basics. 10
2. Sleep Needs 29
3. Sleep Hygiene 36
4. Sleep Safety. 55

Part 2: Sleep Disorders
1. Signs and Symptoms of Sleep Disorders 68
2. Treatment of Sleep Disorders 78

Part 3: Step-by-Step Guide to Better Sleep
1. Childhood Insomnia (Sleeplessness). 88
2. Nocturnal Eating (Drinking) Syndrome. 94
3. Sleep-Onset Association Disorder 106
4. Limit-Setting Disorder. 125
5. Circadian Rhythm Sleep Disorders
   (Delayed and Advanced Sleep Phase Syndrome) 132
6. Excessive Crying 149
7. Confusional Arousals, Night Terrors,
   and Sleepwalking. 158
8. Nightmares and Nighttime Anxiety 168
9. Snoring, Apnea, and Hypoventilation 178
10. Bed-Wetting (Enuresis). 192
11. Restless Legs Syndrome 199
12. Teeth Grinding and Gnashing (Bruxism). 208
13. Rhythmic Movement Disorder 213
14. Narcolepsy. 218
15. Teenage Sleepiness 226
16. Sleep During Pregnancy 235

Better Sleep Resources 242
References 244
Acknowledgments. 251
Index 252

Contributors

Mark Feldman, MD, FRCPC
(Part 3, Chapter 10)
Assistant Professor of Paediatrics,
Consultant, Ambulatory Paediatrics,
Department of Paediatrics,
The Hospital for Sick Children and
University of Toronto
Chief, Department of Paediatrics,
Saint Joseph's Health Centre, Toronto

James MacFarlane, BSc, MSc, PhD
(Part 1, Chapter 1)
Diplomate of the American Board of
Sleep Medicine
Assistant Professor of Paediatrics and
Psychiatry, Department of Paediatrics,
The Hospital for Sick Children and
University of Toronto
Lab Director, Centre for Sleep &
Chronobiology, Toronto

Ian B. MacLusky, MBBS, FRCPC
(Part 3, Chapter 9)
Associate Professor of Paediatrics,
Division of Respiratory Medicine,
Department of Paediatrics,
Director, Pulmonary and Sleep
Laboratories, The Hospital for Sick
Children and University of Toronto

Golda Milo-Manson, MHSc, MD, FRCPC
(Part 2, Chapter 2)
Assistant Professor of Paediatrics,
Division of Developmental Paediatrics,
The Hospital for Sick Children and
University of Toronto
Chief of Medical Staff, Bloorview Kids
Rehab, Toronto

Eileen P. Sloan, MD, PhD, FRCPC
(Part 3, Chapter 16)
Assistant Professor of Psychiatry,
Department of Psychiatry, Mount Sinai
Hospital and University of Toronto
Psychiatrist, Centre for Sleep &
Chronobiology, Toronto

Robyn Stremler, RN, PhD
(Part 3, Chapter 6 and 8)
Assistant Professor, Faculty of Nursing,
Clinician Scientist, The Hospital for Sick
Children and University of Toronto

Introduction

I F YOU HAVE PROBLEMS with getting your baby, toddler, school-aged child, or teenager to sleep at night (or in the case of teenagers, getting them to wake up in the morning), you are not alone. Many parents have concerns about their children's sleep, no matter the age of their child. Research studies tell us that approximately 25% of all children experience some type of sleep problem. Even though some of these problems are not disruptive, severe, or long-lasting, others may result in significant consequences for your child's daytime behavior, family function, and academic performance. Your child's sleep problems may also have a significant impact on your sleep. Coping with multiple sleepless nights while caring for or worrying about your child is not easy, to say the least. Sleepless parents can quickly become as irritable as their sleepless children.

Thankfully, there are many ways to prevent and treat sleep problems in children. In addition to speaking to your child's medical doctor or nurse, you can read about sleep problems in various parenting magazines and numerous books on this topic. There is also a world of collective wisdom concerning children's sleep — every grandparent, friend, neighbor, and co-worker seems ready to offer advice based on their personal experience. However, much of this information, including that offered by the experts, is confusing. Our book is designed to dispel confusion about sleep problems by offering you the best information on children's sleep available, based on recent scientific research and our extensive clinical experience at The Hospital for Sick Children.

We have written this book for expectant parents who want to prevent childhood sleep problems, as well as for parents who want to solve existing sleep difficulties in their children. How you expect your child to sleep is ultimately your choice, based on your own sleep experiences, cultural influences, parenting style, and knowledge of sleep in children. There is no single correct method to improve sleep in children in all families, but some methods are more effective than others for establishing healthy sleep habits and for restoring healthy sleep once it has been disrupted.

> Our book is designed to dispel confusion about sleep problems by offering you the best information on children's sleep available, based on recent scientific research and our extensive clinical experience at The Hospital for Sick Children.

Better Sleep for Your Baby & Child is divided into three sections. In Part 1, we present basic information on healthy sleep, answering such questions as, What is sleep? and How much sleep does my child need? We present preventive strategies for good sleep hygiene and discuss the various options for sleep arrangements, including sleeping with your infant in your own room. In Part 2, we describe various sleep disorders as they occur through the ages, from birth to adolescence, and introduce behavioral and drug treatment strategies. In Part 3, we provide a step-by-step guide to treating specific sleep disorders, ranging from childhood insomnia and sleepwalking to nightmares and bed-wetting. Although many childhood sleep problems can be solved with a behavioral approach, we indicate when you need to consult your doctor for medical or surgical options for other sleep disorders, such as narcolepsy (medical) or sleep apnea (often surgical).

We trust that the prevention and treatment strategies we recommend will enable your child to establish better sleep habits that will help lay the foundation for lifelong health and well-being.

— *Dr. Shelly K.Weiss, MD*

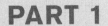

PART 1

Healthy Sleep

CHAPTER 1 Sleep Basics 10

CHAPTER 2 Sleep Needs 29

CHAPTER 3 Sleep Hygiene 36

CHAPTER 4 Sleep Safety 55

Chapter 1

Sleep Basics

THERE'S NOTHING IN the world more peaceful than watching your newborn baby sleep. You can only imagine what your child is dreaming about as she smiles sweetly. There's no greater joy than watching your toddler, who never seems to stop, finally nod off to sleep, restoring his energy for another day of adventure, or admiring your teenager spread across his unmade bed, sound asleep after a day at the beach.

However, there are few things more disturbing to our sense of being a good parent than the distress of sleep problems in our children. This can occur at any age, from trying to comfort a sleepless baby who you know just needs to get some sleep, to dealing with a sleep-deprived adolescent who argues with you until you are worn down about why his activity schedule does not leave time for sleep.

To understand why and how your child sleeps, let's turn to the textbooks. Sleep specialists have studied the biology of sleep for many years now. Their discoveries will help you not only to understand the basics of sleep but also to use this knowledge for improving your child's sleep so that everyone in the family sleeps better, wakes easier, and functions better during the daytime. If you suspect your child has a serious sleep problem, these same basics will help you describe the symptoms to your doctor and cooperate in any recommended treatments. In this case, a little bit of knowledge does go a long way.

What Is Sleep?

Sleep is a reversible state, where you have reduced responsiveness to your environment and minimal movement. Sleep is as essential to our well-being as food and water. We cannot survive without sleep. When you are deprived of sleep, you will become ill and may die. However, we are not sure exactly how sleep sustains and refreshes us. Beyond this life-sustaining role, what are the functions of sleep?

We can infer the functions of sleep based on what happens to us when we don't get enough sleep. Sleep offers more than a time to rest our body and our brain, though this regenerative or

---

Did You Know?

Sleep Health and Distress
Healthy sleep is a source of parental pride and pleasure. If your child is not sleeping well, however, this can lead to difficulty functioning during the day for your child and for you, anxiety about the general health of your child, conflict in your marriage, and a host of other personal and family problems.

Probable Functions of Sleep

- Restoration and regeneration of body systems
- Protection and recovery from infections
- Consolidation of memory
- Optimum daytime function of learning, memory, mood, attention, and concentration
- Growth and development of body and brain

case study: **Sarah**

Jerome and Claire brought their 2-month-old infant Sarah to our sleep clinic. Claire is nursing Sarah about every 3 to 4 hours on demand, and although she is gaining weight well, Jerome and Claire have some concerns. Sarah seems to have her days and nights mixed up, being more wakeful during the night. This is tolerable for now, but Claire has to return to work in 1 month and does not know how she will cope. She wants to continue to nurse Sarah, but needs to get some sleep.

Jerome and Claire have also noticed that Sarah has some funny movements, including making funny faces, sometimes smiling, sometimes grimacing, and often twitching during sleep. They have not noticed this activity at all when she is awake. They are quite concerned that this movement is not normal, but are not sure what is causing it. To alleviate Jerome and Claire's concerns about Sarah, we gave them a quick course in sleep basics. Sarah is thriving, but apparently has not yet developed a circadian pattern to her sleep. That's why her days and nights are mixed up. This is a normal pattern for a newborn up to the age of 3 months. The movements they describe sound normal. Learning about the different stages of sleep and what happens in each stage will help Jerome and Claire to understand that they are probably watching Sarah during the dreaming phase of sleep. Jerome and Claire can rest easy knowing that Sarah, too, is resting normally. Her grimacing, smiling, and twitching at night are part of her normal dreaming sleep pattern.

Over the next few months, soon after Claire had returned to work, they were able to change their interactions with Sarah, playing with her more during the day and decreasing playtime during the night. She began to sleep more at night by 4 months of age.

restorative function is vital. We all know that a lack of sleep affects our memory, mood, attention, and concentration adversely. When you miss a night of sleep, you are probably grouchy and irritable the next day. Imagine how it will affect your child if he is getting less sleep than needed on a constant basis.

Less obviously, poor sleep reduces our ability to deal with serious infections. When our body fights an infection or has some repair work to do (in response to a sunburn, for example), the immune system releases substances to promote sleep and ensure rest. Especially important in children, disturbed sleep can disrupt long-term physical and mental growth. Approximately 75% of brain growth occurs after birth. Healthy sleep is thought to be important for this growth.

Did You Know?

Growth Hormone
All growth in children occurs during sleep. Growth hormone is released from the pituitary gland in the brain while a child sleeps. If something prevents normal sleep on a long-term basis, growth and development may slow down or even stop. All children grow slightly during sleep, and shrink slightly while awake. Fortunately, children grow more than they shrink, but, in extreme cases of poor quality or quantity of sleep, the rate of growth can be adversely influenced.

Sleep States

It seems obvious, but how do we really know when someone is sleeping? Can you tell just from looking at someone if she is truly sleeping? When we sleep, are we in one continuous sleep state? When we sleep, there are important changes in our behavior, body functions, and brain activity that are different from the waking state.

Behavioral Changes

When you are asleep, you do not respond to stimulation in the same way as when you are awake. At times when your baby is sleeping, he is deeply asleep and no amount of noise will wake him, but at other times, it seems like the sound of your whisper across the room easily rouses him. This is because not all sleep is the same. During some of the sleep stages, we can be aroused easily, and during others, we seem to be able to sleep through anything. This is important for deciding what type of sleep problem your child may be experiencing. For example, if your child is experiencing a nightmare, he awakens easily, but if he is in the midst of sleepwalking, it will be difficult to wake him.

Physical Changes

When we fall asleep, the body functions somewhat differently than when we are awake. If you watch your sleeping child, you will notice that there are two different types of sleep. For example, when your child is in the resting state of sleep, you may notice that his breathing rate and heart rate are slow and steady. His eyes do not move rapidly beneath his closed eyelids in this state, which is why it is called non-rapid eye movement sleep, or NREM sleep. When your child is in the dreaming state of sleep, you may notice that his muscle tone is decreased so that, other than some muscle twitches, he has little movement. In this dreaming state, his breathing rate and heart rate will be irregular,

Q. What is a brain wave?

A. The nerve cells (called neurons) in the brain produce electrical signals, which can be captured and displayed as brain waves. These brain waves change, depending on the activity of the nerve cells in the brain. During REM sleep, the waves resemble waking brain waves because your brain in this stage of sleep is active. During NREM sleep, the waves are slower, which reflects that your brain is in a resting stage.

and you may see bursts of eye movement under his eyelids. This is called rapid eye movement sleep, or REM sleep. Scientists who study sleep monitor these changes in awake and sleep states by analyzing heart rate, breathing rate, muscle tone, eye movements, and brain waves.

Brain Changes

Sleep is not simply the absence of wakefulness, and not all sleep is the same. During the night, your child moves in and out of sleep states in a predictable way. If you wait 10 to 20 minutes after your child first falls asleep, you can change his pajamas, move him, or make lots of noise and he will continue to sleep. This is because soon after falling asleep, he is in a stage of deep sleep, from which he is less likely to arouse. At other times, your child appears restless, moving, and may talk in his sleep. While we do have a diminished conscious awareness of our surroundings during sleep, there are times during sleep, especially while we are dreaming, when our brain is as active or, occasionally, more active than when we are awake.

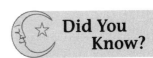

Did You Know?

REM Facts
Infants and children spend a greater percentage of their sleep in the REM stage. In fact, newborns spend 50% of their sleep in REM sleep. This gradually decreases to 20% to 25% as an adult. REM sleep is thought to be important for consolidating learning and memory in children.

SLEEP STATES

REM: Rapid eye movement sleep or dreaming sleep. Although REM is commonly referred to as dreaming sleep, you dream during all stages of sleep, but dreams are more vivid and complex during REM sleep.

NREM: Non-rapid eye movement sleep

Four Stages of NREM Sleep
The four stages (1 to 4) of NREM sleep go from the lightest (stage 1) to the deepest (stage 4) of sleep.

Stage 1: Transitional sleep or light NREM sleep
This stage is called transitional because it is the stage of sleep through which children (after the first 3 months of age) and adults transition from wake to sleep when feeling drowsy.

Stage 2: Medium NREM sleep
This stage can be thought of as the 'glue of sleep' as it is the stage in which both children and adults spend almost one-half of their sleeping time. Like glue, this stage is important for holding together the pattern or 'architecture' of sleep.

Stages 3 and 4: Deep NREM sleep or slow-wave sleep
These are the most restful, restorative phases of sleep.

NREM and REM Sleep States

There are two different states of sleep: NREM and REM sleep. During the night, we cycle in a predicable way from one state to another, between NREM and REM sleep. When we change from one sleep state to another, we may have a brief period of waking, called an arousal. If the arousal is brief, then we just move to the

REM versus NREM Sleep

	NREM Sleep	REM Sleep
Function of this state	Transitional and restful, restorative stage of sleep	Most dreaming (especially dreams we are able to remember) takes place; thought to be important for formation of memory
Ability to move muscles	All muscles are more relaxed than in the awake state but still able to move	All muscles are relaxed, almost paralyzed except for muscles controlling eye movement, hearing, and breathing
Movement	Able to turn over, change position in bed	Muscle twitches, facial grimaces, and sounds related to dreaming
Eye movement	No rapid eye movement	Bursts of rapid eye movement
Breathing rate	Breathing rate is more regular If you watch your child, you will notice steady breathing	Breathing rate is more irregular If your child has sleep apnea, he will have more episodes during this phase when he has decreased muscle tone
Brain activity	Brain activity shows slowing of function into four stages from stage 1 (drowsy) to stage 4 (deepest) stage with most slowing of activity	Brain waves look similar to when awake Your child's brain uses the same amount of oxygen as when he is awake
Time of night (sleep cycle)	The deepest stage of sleep (slow-wave sleep stages 3 and 4) is in the first one-third of the night Children may have another episode of deep sleep in the early morning	Most REM sleep is in the last one-third of the night
Ability to be woken from sleep	Easy to be aroused in lighter stages 1 and 2 Hardest to be aroused in deeper stages 3 and 4	Easy to be aroused

SLEEP HYPNOGRAM

This chart of sleep states, called a sleep hypnogram, shows a normal sleep pattern for a child during one night of sleep. This predictable sleep pattern is called sleep architecture, and should be quite stable from one night to the next.

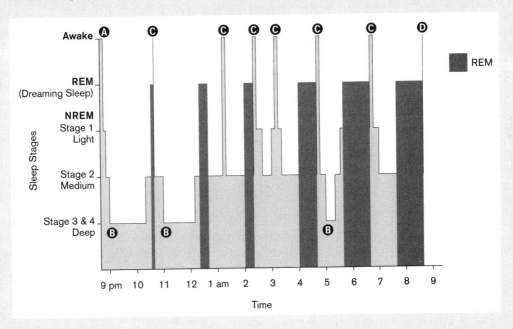

A Your child typically falls asleep quickly, in less than 30 minutes. Transitional sleep is brief and easily reversed.

B Your child will quickly have her first episode of deep sleep, and continue to have her most deep sleep in the first one-third of the night. Your child may have a briefer episode of deep restorative sleep in the early morning hours before waking.

C There may be periods of brief arousal during the night. When your child ends one sleep cycle and starts the next, he may have a brief period of awakening. These arousals occur out of the REM or the lighter stages of NREM sleep. In normal sleep, your child will not remember these episodes in the morning.

D Your child should wake up spontaneously in the morning.

Dreaming Sleep: The first episode of dreaming sleep happens about 1½ hours after falling asleep. The dreaming episodes become longer throughout the night, with most dreaming happening in the last one-third of the night.

Sleep Cycles: Your child will cycle from dreaming (REM) to restorative sleep (NREM) throughout the night. The cycles lengthen with development. At 1 year of age, the cycle may last 45 to 50 minutes, and at age 5 to10 years, the cycle lengthens to 60 to 70 minutes. The cycles continue to lengthen with growth to adult levels of 90 to 110 minutes.

next sleep stage, and in the morning, we do not remember being awake or feel any adverse effects of this normal arousal. If the arousal is longer (lasting more than a few seconds), then we experience a short period of waking, and, whether or not we remember it, it may cause daytime fatigue.

Regulating the Sleep/Wake Cycle

How do you regulate your baby's sleep/wake cycle so that he is awake during the day and sleeping at night? What helps him get enough sleep to feel well rested during the day? There are two processes that work together to regulate sleep and wake, called process S and process C. These processes help us to sleep at the right time and to ensure that we get an adequate amount of sleep.

Process S

The longer your child goes without sleep, the stronger will be her drive to fall asleep. If the pressure to sleep is great enough, she may not be able to maintain wakefulness and become drowsy and even fall asleep in a dangerous situation. This can lead to motor vehicle accidents if your teenager is sleep-deprived and becomes drowsy while driving. The longer we go without sleep, the deeper and longer we will sleep to catch up. If, for example, your teenager gets less sleep than required several nights of the week, staying up late to work, study, or socialize, and waking up early to get to school, when the weekend comes, he is able to sleep for 12 or more hours because process S is pulling him to try and catch up on his sleep debt.

Process C

The other important regulator of sleep is called the circadian process, or process C. This is the biological clock that sets the daily pattern of sleep and waking and other activities that recur about every 24 hours. Our natural sleep/wake schedule is a bit longer than 24 hours, so each day we need to reset our biological clock by using internal and external biological cues to stay on a 24-hour day cycle. These cues are called zeitgebers (from the German — zeit:time; geber:giver). Newborn infants are not born with a functioning rhythmical (circadian) process and initially sleep and wake on an erratic schedule. As they develop, gaining the ability to respond to internal and external cues over the first few months of life, they are able to develop a more mature schedule that resembles yours, sleeping longer at night and being more awake during the day.

ZEITGEBERS (CIRCADIAN CUES)

Can you imagine what life would be like if you lived in a dark world without sunlight or structure, and you had no commitments forcing you to wake up each day at the same time to get to work or school? It would be hard for you to maintain a 24-hour day-night schedule because of the lack of zeitgebers, or cues to your circadian rhythm. Zeitgebers are the time cues that keep our biological clock working on a 24-hour day. These signals are relayed through complex pathways in the brain to adjust our biological clocks constantly and affect our daily rhythms, including the release of hormones, such as cortisol, growth hormone, and melatonin, as well as the regulation of metabolism and body temperature, which all have unique timing in relation to the sleep/wake cycle.

Light/Dark: Sunlight is the most important cue to the circadian rhythms to keep us functioning on a 24-hour cycle. Take, for example, two different 12-year-old children, who wake up differently on Saturday morning. Eliza wakes up at 8:00 a.m. and drags her blanket into the den, where the curtains are tightly shut, and turns on cartoons. She lies on the couch in the darkened room and watches television, half asleep, until 11:00 when the rest of the family wakens. At 11:00, she eats breakfast in another room with the bright morning light streaming in. Another child, Madeline, wakes up on Saturday morning at 8:00 a.m., and takes her dog outside for a walk in the sunshine. She returns after 20 minutes, and, hungry from the exercise, sits down to eat breakfast. Which child will have an easier time falling asleep on Saturday night? Although Eliza and Madeline woke up at the same time, because Eliza rests without natural light until 11:00 a.m., her biological clock didn't receive this cue until then. Madeline provided her clock with the most important cue — light exposure early in the morning.

In addition to the importance of being exposed to sunlight in the morning, it is also important to sleep in a darkened room, another cue signaling the biological clock that it is now night and time to rest. A night-light or a dim hall or closet light left on through the night is fine, provided the bedroom is dark.

Meal Timing: Eating breakfast in the morning at a regular time is another cue to the body that it is morning. At the end of the day, it is important to avoid heavy meals when the body is ready to rest. This prevents your stomach from being busy digesting food when you are trying to sleep.

Social Activities: Another cue to our biological clock is a social cue. We are motivated to be awake in the morning and sleep at night by school, work, and social schedules. For example, if you have an early morning meeting, you know that you should get to sleep at a time that will give you enough hours of sleep to be refreshed in the morning. Children who are developmentally delayed may lack this motivation and do not have this cue to help keep their internal clocks working properly.

Environmental Temperature: There is a natural rhythm to our core temperature, which is at its lowest when we are sleeping in the early morning hours. If the bedroom temperature at night is too hot or too cold, this adversely affects our ability to sleep and keep our biological clock working properly. Therefore, you want your child's room (and your own bedroom) to be at a comfortable cool temperature at night. This will be the temperature at which an adult who is lightly clothed would be comfortable.

Noise: Another important cue to keep our sleep/wake cycle on a 24-hour day schedule is quiet at night and noise in the day. For example, when your infant wakes at night and needs to be fed or changed, try to do so as quietly as possible to reinforce the difference between night and day. It is not necessary for you to make lots of noise during the day to keep your baby awake, just a reasonable amount will let him know it is time to be awake.

What Is Normal Sleep?

We know that our tendency or desire to sleep at different times of the day changes in a predictable way with age. For example, if you and your teenage daughter decide to attend a lecture in the evening at 9:00 p.m, who would have more difficulty staying awake? The answer is that your teenager (like most teenagers) will likely be much more alert than you (his parents) in the evening. Don't you remember being more alert in the evening when you were a teenager?

What if you were asked to give the lecture and to choose the time to deliver it? If your goal is to have your audience wide awake and listening to you speak, you would not choose to give a lecture right after lunch in the early afternoon. No matter what our age, this is the time of day when our tendency to sleep is very high (like in the early morning before sunrise), whereas we are less likely to be sleepy later in the morning.

These alert/drowsy times change as your child grows from infancy to adolescence. For example, a school-age child will have a strong desire to sleep in the late evening hours, but a teenager will not have the same biological drive to sleep at this time. The timing of sleep tendency is determined by process C. The magnitude of this tendency is determined by process S.

Fetal Sleep Patterns

It is remarkable what scientists can tell us about sleep even before birth. Babies show clear sleep/wake patterns from about the sixth month of pregnancy onward. Researchers have shown

AVERAGE SLEEP REQUIREMENTS FROM BIRTH THROUGH ADULTHOOD

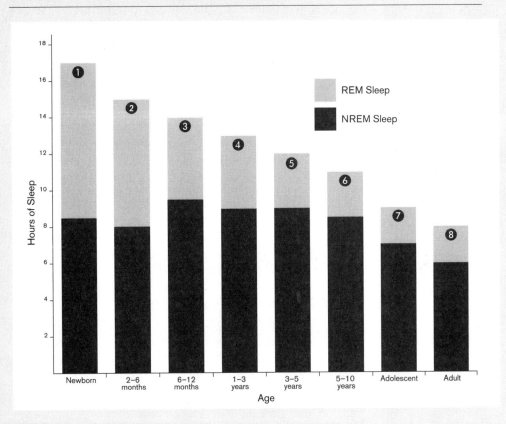

This graph shows a gradual decrease in the average amount of sleep required from birth through adolescence. It also shows the percentages of REM and NREM sleep and how they change at each stage of life.

Bars

1 *Newborn (0 to 2 months)*
Average sleep: 16 to 18 hours
REM: 50%

2 *Infant (2 to 6 months)*
Average sleep: 14 to 16 hours
REM: less than 50%

3 *Infant (6 to 12 months)*
Average sleep: 13 to 15 hours
REM: decreases to 30% by
12 months

4 *Toddler (1 to 3 years)*
Average sleep: 12 to 14 hours
REM: 25% to 30%

5 *Preschooler (3 to 5 years)*
Average sleep: 11 to 13 hours
REM: decreased to 25% by 5 years

6 *School Age (5 to 10 years)*
Average sleep: 10 to 11 hours
REM: 20% to 25%

7 *Early-late Adolescence*
Average sleep: 8.5 to 9.5 hours
REM: 20% to 25%

8 *Young Adult*
Average sleep: 8 hours
REM: 20% to 25%

clear activity-rest cycles that, to some extent, follow the mother's activity-rest cycle. During the last 2 months of pregnancy until your baby is born, the sleep cycles develop so that we see clear evidence for periods of wake, periods of quiet sleep (early form of NREM) sleep, and periods of active sleep (early form of REM or dreaming sleep). What does a fetus dream about? We can only guess.

Newborn Sleep Patterns (0–3 Months)

Newborn babies are beautiful human beings, perfect in every way except, you might say, for their newborn sleep-wake cycles. Newborns sleep and wake without regard for day or night. From the moment of birth, we all know too well that the sleep-wake cycle of a newborn is very different from the rest of the family's.

Newborns need much more sleep than an older child, teenager, or adult. Most newborns sleep between 16 and 18 out of 24 hours. Newborns will usually sleep after 60 to 120 minutes of wakefulness, and each sleep period will be for 2 to 4 hours. You should look for signs of drowsiness in your baby and help him fall asleep after he has been awake for this amount of time.

Newborns also have no ability to regulate when they sleep. Babies do not regulate their sleep and wake to the day-night cycle, but rather they will wake when they are hungry, and sleep when their tummy is full or when they are tired. This unusual sleep-wake pattern is normal for the first few months of life. The best thing for the baby's mother to do, though not always possible, is to sleep when her baby sleeps, so both mother and child are getting as much rest as possible.

Sleep and Development

During this period of your newborn's life, sleep and brain development are closely related, particularly development of your child's biological clock:

Brain Development

The brain develops so that sleep stages can be clearly recognized. During the first 3 months of life, there is rapid development of your baby's brain, which is reflected in changes that you see in every aspect of his life. Some of these changes are seen in his social development, such as smiling and becoming more social, and some changes are seen in his motor skills, such as holding up his head and gaining control over other body muscles. Other

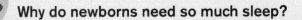

Q. **Why do newborns need so much sleep?**

A. Half of your baby's sleep will be in the dreaming state and half in the non-dreaming state. During the 8 hours a day that your baby spends in dreaming sleep, his brain is growing and developing at an astonishing rate. Sleep scientists hypothesize that dream sleep stimulates brain growth and development, which is important for learning and memory formation. However, your baby also needs to spend about 8 hours a day in non-dreaming sleep. This part of sleep is responsible for body growth. These are just two important reasons why your baby needs so much sleep.

changes are reflected in his sleep patterns. By the age of 3 months, a baby will develop some of the brain-wave patterns seen during sleep that reflect further brain development. This timing of brain development and the beginning of more mature sleep patterns are both seen simultaneously at about 3 months of age.

Biological Clock

Your baby's internal biological clock begins to recognize signals, which help him to sleep longer periods at night instead of randomly sleeping day or night. The timing of an infant's sleep is also very different in the first 3 months of life. Your newborn baby will have no preference for the longer sleep periods at night. By 3 months of age, due to the ongoing maturation of the brain and the influence of cues or signals to the brain about day and night, he will begin to develop a new sleep pattern, where he can have longer sleep periods during the night and shorter sleep periods during the day. The cues are social, from interacting more during the day than at night, and biological, from his ability to develop a rhythm based on the light-dark cycle of day and night.

Q. **How do we know when a baby is dreaming?**

A. Your baby will have these signs: sucking, fine twitches, tremors, grimaces, smiles, and intermittent stretching and movements of the limbs. If you watch your baby sleep and see some of these signs, you will know he is dreaming.

Infant Sleep Patterns

3 to 6 Months

Although your baby's brain matures rapidly and changes do occur in his sleep by 3 months of age, up until about the age of 6 months, the part of the brain that controls the timing of sleep is not fully developed. So, your baby develops the ability to control this sleep-wake cycle during the first 6 months of life.

During this time, an infant's waking, sleeping, and feeding are done in a rather random fashion. In fact, the sleep-wake pattern is almost entirely driven by the repeated need for feeding during these first few months. Sleep researchers are studying whether you can start to change these patterns during these early months. However, it is already known that from 3 to 6 months of age, you can start to make changes to the signals that you give your baby to help lengthen nighttime sleep. Some babies can settle on their own, even as infants. If you need to help your baby to fall asleep, you can help him establish good sleep habits by slowly decreasing the nurturing (feeding, cuddling, rocking) that helps him fall asleep and by putting him in bed drowsy but awake. You can also let natural light into the room in the morning and keep the room dark at night, using only a night-light when changing or feeding him at night.

6 to 12 Months

By the time your baby is 6 months old, she has developed rapidly in many ways. Some developmental skills are easy to recognize, such as an incredible increase in muscle strength. A newborn cannot support her own head, but by 6 months, your baby is already learning to sit. Other growth is not so readily visible, notably maturation of the brain cells that control sleep and allow your child to develop a more mature sleep-wake pattern.

At approximately 6 to 8 months, the brain center that controls the timing of sleep is finally working, and your baby will slowly begin to synchronize with the schedules of the family. Your baby will start to sleep for longer periods during the night and wake for longer periods during the day. Infants will typically continue to have two naps during the day. Of course, these are all welcomed stages of development for helping you and your family to create some routines.

By 9 months of age, 70% to 80% of infants will sleep through the night (which will be at least 6 hours at a time). Your baby will be able to go for longer periods between feedings, which explains the longer sleep periods. Your baby in every way will begin to respond more and more to all sources of stimulation in the environment that you provide.

Average Sleep

- At 3 months, an infant's average sleep is 14 to 16 hours per 24 hours.
- At 6 months, an infant's average sleep is 13 to 15 hours per 24 hours.

Average Sleep

- At 6 to 12 months, your baby's average sleep is 13 to 15 hours per 24 hours, more or less.
- In a study of 500 healthy children at 6 months, parents reported that 50% slept between 13 and 15.5 hours; 25% slept between 10.5 and 13 hours; and 25% slept between 15.5 and 18 hours a day.
- In a study of 500 healthy children at 12 months, parents reported that 50% slept between 13 and 15 hours; 25% slept between 11.5 and 13 hours; and 25% slept between 15 and 16.5 hours.

TYPICAL SLEEP/WAKE PATTERN AT 9 MONTHS

Bedtime: 6:30 to 7:30 p.m.

Sleep at night: 10 to 12 hours (maybe interrupted by brief wakings)

Wake time: 6:00 to 7:00 a.m.

First nap: 2 to 3 hours after waking

Second nap: 2 to 3 hours after waking from first nap

Third nap: By 6 to 12 months of age, most babies will decrease the number of daytime naps from 3 to 2

Toddler Sleep Patterns

The sleep-wake cycle continues to develop so that by the time your baby is 2 years old, this pattern should be well developed. Between 1 and 3 years of age, your child now requires about 12 hours of sleep a day. You may be getting up with your toddler at night (like many parents with children of this age), but this is probably now just a habit that you and your child have developed. We know that babies can learn to sleep through the night around 6 months of age, and definitely by the age of 2 years. Your toddler also has the capacity to learn to do this. At this age, sleep should

Q. **When should afternoon naps be discontinued?**

A. There is no definite age when your child should give up her afternoon nap. It depends on your child. If your child is at daycare and all the other children nap in the afternoon, she will likely continue this pattern until she graduates from day care and starts school. However, if your child happens to be enrolled in an afternoon preschool, nursery, or kindergarten program, then she will have to give up her afternoon nap, maybe even earlier than you would have chosen. She may then adopt a schedule with one longer nighttime sleep episode.

The best way to know if your child is ready to give up her nap is to watch how she does during the day and if it takes her longer than 30 minutes to fall asleep at naptime. Notice if she seems well rested. There can be many causes why children have trouble with behavior, attention span, or playing with peers, but remember that one possibility in your toddler and preschooler may be that she is not getting enough sleep and needs longer sleep at night or a regular afternoon nap.

TYPICAL SLEEP/WAKE PATTERN FOR A YOUNGER TODDLER WITH ONE AFTERNOON NAP

Bedtime: 7:00 to 8:00 p.m.

Sleep at night: 10 to 12 hours

Wake time: 6:00 to 7:00 a.m.

Afternoon nap: 12:00 to 1:00 p.m. (1 to 3 hours)

Average Sleep

- At 1 to 3 years of age, your toddler's average sleep is 12 to 14 hours per 24 hours, more or less.
- In a study of 500 healthy children at 3 years of age, parents reported that 50% slept between 12 and 14 hours; 25% slept from 10.5 to 12 hours; and 25% slept from 14 to 15 hours.

Average Sleep

- At 3 to 5 years of age, your child's average sleep is 11 to 13 hours per 24 hours.

be continuous at night. However, your toddler will still require a nap (usually in the afternoon) so her sleep will occur in two phases — an afternoon nap and nighttime sleep.

This is pattern is very natural. In fact, adults in many cultures maintain this pattern of two sleep cycles a day — one short sleep in the afternoon and one longer sleep episode at night. For most adults living in North America, the afternoon nap is no longer possible given work schedules.

Your toddler's sleep patterns will also be changed when she learns to climb out of her crib and starts to sleep in a child- or adult-size bed. This may present new challenges if you are having trouble getting her to sleep at night or to stay in bed.

Preschool Sleep Patterns

Most children between 3 and 5 years will consolidate the nap and night sleep into one continuous sleep period at night. However, a few children will continue to have an afternoon nap until starting school around the age of 6 years. Until adolescence, this pattern will remain constant 7 days a week. There is no sleeping-in on the weekends for your child, and probably not for you. Children tend to wake at the same time each day, and this is why it is important to try and have bedtime also at the same time each night.

TYPICAL SLEEP/WAKE PATTERN FOR A PRESCHOOLER WITHOUT AN AFTERNOON NAP

Bedtime: 7:00 to 8:00 p.m.

Nighttime sleep: 11 to 13 hours

Wake time: 6:00 to 7:00 a.m.

Child Sleep Patterns

By the time your child is 6 years old, sleep is as perfect as it will ever get. Children between ages 6 and 12 years should fall asleep rapidly and stay asleep throughout the night. Sleep is consolidated into one sleep episode at night. There should be no need for napping during the day. Children at this age may not have this well-developed, healthy sleep/wake pattern if there are sleep problems that started prior to school age.

Sleep Pattern Changes

- Now similar to the adult sleep pattern
- About 50% of the night is spent in medium NREM sleep
- About 25% is spent in deep NREM sleep
- About 25% is spent in dreaming (REM) sleep

Adolescent Sleep Patterns

The pattern of sleep in teenagers is similar to that of adults. There is a decrease in deep slow-wave (stage 3 and 4 NREM) sleep from the age of 5 to 15, with a concurrent increase in the amount of lighter stages of NREM sleep. The amount and timing of sleep changes for a variety of reasons.

Aging

As your child grows from a child to a teenager, less sleep is needed in most cases.

New Demands

Teenagers experience more academic demands, become more involved in extracurricular activities, take on part-time employment, and regularly socialize with friends — all contributing to less time for sleep.

Inadequate Sleep

Many teenagers obtain less sleep than is required. Although the duration of sleep that is needed, between 8.5 and 9.5 hours of sleep according to research, does not change significantly between 12 and 18 years, many studies show that teenagers (on average) usually get less sleep. Research also shows that older adolescents are sleepier during the daytime than younger adolescents.

Average Sleep
- At 6 to 12 years, your child will sleep approximately 10 to 11 hours per night, gradually declining to just over 9 hours per night by age 12.

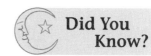
Did You Know?

Fewer Dreams
The change in required sleep from newborn to age 12 is almost entirely due to the reduction in the need for dreaming sleep. A newborn may spend 8 to 9 hours a day in dreaming sleep, which decreases to $2\frac{1}{4}$ hours for a 12-year-old. This change parallels the development of the brain and acquisition of many of the most complex behaviors that we must learn (for example, walking and talking).

Parental Involvement

Parents generally become less involved in the bedtime of teenagers and more involved in ensuring that teenagers rise in the morning. This is compounded by the next development of adolescent sleep patterns — sleeping in.

Sleeping In

Teenagers tend to go to sleep later and wake up later on non-school days. There is both a biological and social reason for this change once puberty begins. The biological change is a lengthening of the internal clock, which makes teenagers less sleepy at night, preferring to be 'owl types' who stay up later at night. The social reason for this change is the demands on many teenagers such as, homework, part-time jobs, extracurricular, and sporting activities, in addition to using the telephone, Internet, television, and video games in the evening.

Irregular Patterns

Teenagers tend to have a larger difference between their sleep schedules on school days and non-school days. Bedtime and waking times become delayed (except on school mornings). A pattern develops where there is a large discrepancy between the time of sleep onset and rise time between school nights and weekends. In some school districts, teenagers have to start school earlier in high school than in middle school.

Sleep Disturbances

Teenagers may use substances that impact the onset of sleep and sleep continuity. Substances that may be used or abused by some teenagers, such as nicotine, caffeine, alcohol, and nonprescription drugs, all have the ability to cause significant sleep disturbances.

Sleep Questions

Although considerable research has been directed to studying how we sleep and why we may not sleep well, there are still many things we do not know about sleep, including children's sleep. For example:

- We believe that by treating sleep problems in childhood, we will prevent sleep problems as adults, but this theory has not been scientifically tested.
- We do not know what (if any) the long-term consequences are of successfully treating sleep problems in childhood.

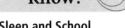

Did You Know?

Sleep and School
Research studies show that teenagers with less of a difference in the timing of bed and wake times on school days and non-school days obtain better academic scores, showing the association between sleep regularity and academic success.

SLEEP CHANGES FROM AGE 5 TO 85

This graph was recently published by sleep experts who reviewed all the available studies of normal sleep and then combined the data to make this summary of how sleep changes from the ages of 5 to 85 years. Each stage of sleep and wakefulness during the night is shown separately.

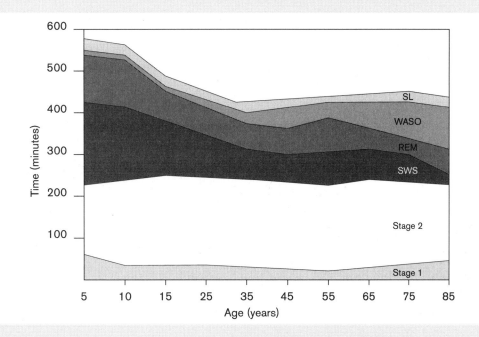

1. **SL (sleep latency):** This is shown on the top line of the graph. Sleep latency means the time it takes you to fall asleep once you are in bed and the lights are out. As you can see, the sleep latency is similar throughout life in healthy children and adults.

2. **WASO:** "Wake after sleep onset" is a measure of how much time you spend awake between the time you first fall asleep and wake up in the morning. You will notice that from 5 to 10 years of age, children sleep most of the night and are awake very little. The amount of time spent in waking state through the night increases in adults compared to children and teenagers.

3. **REM (rapid eye movement sleep or dreaming sleep):** You can see that children between 5 and 10 years of age have a large amount of dreaming sleep, which then decreases slightly.

4. **SWS (slow-wave sleep):** This is the deep sleep (stage 3 and 4 non-REM) that is so prevalent in childhood. The black bar showing the amount of SWS is quite striking. The amount of slow-wave (deep restorative) sleep decreases from childhood to adulthood and then again markedly decreases in the elderly.

5. **Stage 2 NREM (non-rapid eye movement) sleep:** This is medium deep sleep. You can see that the amount of Stage 2 NREM sleep is fairly constant throughout life and makes up a large part of our sleep.

6. **Stage 1 NREM sleep:** This is transitional sleep. We are in Stage 1 briefly when transitioning from wake to sleep and back, and you can see from the graph that the amount of Stage 1 sleep is fairly constant and makes up a small amount of our nightly sleep.

(Adapted by permission from Ohayon MM, et al. Meta-analysis of quantitative sleep parameters from childhood to old age in healthy individuals: Developing normative sleep values across the human lifespan. Sleep 2004;27(7):1255-73.)

- Most studies that have been done focus on children with difficulty settling at bedtime or trouble sleeping through the night. We need more studies on all the other types of childhood sleep problems.

- There are few studies on the use of medications in treating sleep disorders in children. Therefore, we do not know the exact rationale for using medications, which ones (if any) would be best, and how long to use them.

- There is some research that shows that the hours children sleep may vary from one country to another, but we do not know if children raised in one country need more or less sleep than another.

We do know that different children need different amounts of sleep to feel rested in the morning and to remain alert during the day. But how much sleep does your child need? That is the subject of our next chapter.

Chapter 2

Sleep Needs

THE MOST COMMON question that parents ask sleep specialists is, "How much sleep does my child need?" The answer is simple, but not conclusive. Children need different amounts of sleep depending on their age, and within each age group, your child may sleep more or less than the average, but still be getting enough sleep.

How Much Sleep Does My Child Need?

We know from research studies how much sleep children get on average as they grow. These studies are based on questionnaire surveys of parents in different countries around the world. While the desired average amount of sleep that children need at different ages is known, there are individual children who sleep more or less than average and remain healthy and well rested.

Quick Guide to Average Sleep Needs

You may want to record your child's average sleep duration in comparison with sleep studies of many other children.

Age	Average hours	My child sleeps…
0 to 2 months	16 to 18	_____ hours
2 to 6 months	14 to 16	_____ hours
6 to 12 months	13 to 15	_____ hours
1 to 3 years	12 to 14	_____ hours
3 to 5 years	11 to 13	_____ hours
5 to 12 years	10 to 11	_____ hours
12 to 18 years	8.5 to 9.5	_____ hours

Sleep Adequacy Studies

Research has also revealed other facts about sleep needs in different age groups and in different cultures.

Age Groups

- Infants need the most sleep and their need decreases with age.
- School-age children are the least sleepy during the day and the least likely to nap.
- Preadolescents are the second least sleepy age group.
- Teenagers in mid to late adolescence, even if they are getting the correct amount of sleep at night, are sleepier during the daytime than in childhood or in early adolescence.

Cultural Groups

Studies in several countries, including the United States and Canada, document that teenagers are generally getting less sleep than they need.

Sleep need varies somewhat by where you live. In some countries, children obtain either more or less sleep on average, but we do not know if this is because they need more or less, or if cultural differences in parenting practices dictate different amounts of sleep.

---

case study: Gail

Gail was 4 years old when her parents brought her to our sleep clinic. At that time, she resisted bedtime, which was usually at 8:00 p.m., and by the time she settled down and fell asleep, it was usually 10:00 p.m. Gail attends an afternoon preschool program, and because her mother works from home, she can sleep until 9:00 a.m., therefore getting 11 uninterrupted hours of sleep.

During the day, Gail is a happy, well-adjusted child, but her parents worry that she is not getting enough sleep to stay healthy. After further discussion, it was apparent that Gail was not showing any signs of sleep deprivation. She was sleeping within the average for her age category (between 11 and 13 hours). One of the reasons that Gail was able to get enough sleep (which would not apply to all families) is that her mother works from home, and, therefore, she is able to sleep later in the morning. Gail's parents were reassured to hear that she was getting enough sleep and learned from attending the clinic that the important question is not "How much sleep should my child get?" but rather "What are the signs that my child is not getting adequate sleep?"

How Do I Know If My Child Is Getting Enough Sleep?

For you and your child, a more important question than "How much sleep does my child need?" is "How do I know if my child is getting enough sleep?"

If children show symptoms of being sleepy during the day, they are likely not getting enough sleep, regardless of how their

---

SLEEP CHECKUP GUIDE

Healthy Sleep Signs

If your child is getting enough healthy sleep at night, you will be able to answer yes to the following questions. Check them off.

- ☐ My child falls asleep in less than 20 to 30 minutes of bedtime.

- ☐ My child wakes easily in the morning, at an expected time.

- ☐ My child appears well rested during the day.

- ☐ My child stays awake without taking a nap during the day. (This question only applies to children who have outgrown their daytime nap.)

- ☐ My child stays awake during quiet activities, such as driving in the car or watching television.

Inadequate Sleep Symptoms

However, if your child is not getting enough healthy sleep, you or his teacher will be able to answer yes to the following statements. Check them off.

- ☐ My child has difficulty getting up in the morning.

- ☐ My child falls back asleep after being woken and needs parent to wake again or repeatedly.

- ☐ My child yawns frequently during the day.

- ☐ My child complains of feeling tired.

- ☐ My child prefers to lie down during the day, even if she misses activities with family or friends.

- ☐ My child wants to nap during the day.

- ☐ My child lacks interest, motivation, and attention.

- ☐ My child falls asleep or seems drowsy at school during class or at home during homework.

sleep duration stacks up against the average child. Sleep quantity is not the only factor to be considered. Sleep quality can also play an important role in determining if your child gets enough good sleep. We can approach an answer to this question by determining symptoms of inadequate sleep and poor quality sleep.

Mistaken Symptoms

When adults are sleepy, they generally look fatigued. In adults, it is easy to recognize the symptoms of fatigue, but this is not always true in children. When children are tired, some may look fatigued like an adult, but others may not look sleepy and instead exhibit other symptoms, which are, at times, the apparent opposite of being tired:

- Irritable
- Inattentive
- Hyperactive
- Low tolerance to frustration

These symptoms of inadequate sleep may be misdiagnosed as attention deficit/hyperactivity disorder (ADHD) or a behavioral problem. If your child displays these symptoms, you should first think about his quality and quantity of sleep. Try to determine if he is getting enough sleep or if anything is disturbing his sleep. Is he showing any signs of breathing difficulties at night, which could be the signs of sleep apnea disturbing his sleep? Talk to your doctor about these concerns. If he is getting adequate sleep, without any signs of sleep problems, then you can evaluate with his doctor other causes of these symptoms.

Teenage Symptoms

Teenagers may present different symptoms than adults when they are tired. In a teenager, you may see these symptoms of inadequate sleep:

- Use of excessive caffeine in food or drinks for the stimulant effect
- Problems with memory and learning
- Drowsiness or napping during classes
- Difficulty staying awake in the afternoon

Consequences of Inadequate Sleep

Teenagers suffering from inadequate sleep may experience the following consequences and complications:

- Excessive fatigue, such as falling asleep in non-stimulating activities

- Drop in school performance

- Mood changes

- Drowsy driving motor vehicle accidents

- Reliance on stimulant substances and drugs to stay awake during the day

Q. **How do I know if my teenager is not getting enough sleep?**

A. Inadequate sleep in adolescents can be hard to detect, and the consequences can be severe. To determine if your teenager is sleep deprived, try asking yourself these questions:

- Is my teenager excessively sleepy during the day?

- Has my teenager's school performance decreased?

- Does my teenager have a mood disturbance (which can be both caused by or causing the sleep problems)?

- Has my teenager been involved in motor vehicle accidents and other problems caused by daytime sleepiness?

- Does my teenager rely on stimulants and/or drugs to stay awake during the day?

If you answer yes to any one of these questions, you may want to consult your child's doctor.

What Causes Inadequate Sleep?

The most common cause of sleepiness during the day at any age, for children and for adults, is, simply, inadequate sleep. However, there are other causes to consider, including sleep disruption, an increased need for sleep in some people, and several sleep disorders and syndromes.

Sleep Disruptions

There are specific sleep disorders, medical and psychiatric problems, and side effects of medications that can disrupt sleep and cause daytime sleepiness. Anything that causes your child's sleep to be disrupted at night will cause daytime sleepiness. While there are many reasons for sleep to be disrupted, the most common causes in children are based on problems that are easily resolved with behavioral management.

Common Causes of Nighttime Sleep Disruption

- Obstructive sleep apnea
- Nightmares
- Night terrors and sleepwalking; these sleep disrupters can disturb your sleep but not necessarily your child's sleep
- Environmental factors, such as noise, light in the bedroom
- Drugs, either prescribed or street drugs, including nicotine, alcohol, caffeine
- Medical problems, such as asthma, eczema, seizures

Increased Need for Sleep

There are rare sleep disorders where your child may need extra sleep at night. Medical, psychiatric problems, and medications can also contribute to an increased need for sleep. This is the least common cause of sleepiness during the day, but the most common reason to consult your doctor.

Factors in Need for Extra Sleep

- Illness
- Effect of medications, such as antihistamines used in medicine for allergies, motion sickness, or cold medications
- Depression or other mood or psychiatric disorder
- Narcolepsy (a rare cause of excessive daytime sleepiness)

Other Common Causes of Inadequate Sleep

There are several other common problems that can cause your child to have trouble falling asleep at night, staying asleep, or waking too early in the morning.

Did You Know?

Good Quantity, Poor Quality

If your child has an adequate amount of sleep (quantity), but poor sleep continuity (quality), then he will be tired.

Did You Know?

Good Quality, Poor Quantity

If your child is getting restful sleep (quality), but inadequate amount of sleep (quantity), she may need more sleep than she is obtaining.

Difficulty falling asleep at the beginning of the night:

- Inadequate sleep hygiene: for example, having an irregular schedule and inconsistent sleep habits.

- Sleep-onset association disorder: a problem where your child has not learned to fall asleep without you or certain conditions present at bedtime.

- Limit-setting disorder: includes numerous 'curtain calls' from your child who resists bedtime.

- Delayed sleep phase syndrome: a problem with the timing of sleep and wake, where both are delayed.

Difficulty maintaining sleep through the night:

Sleep-onset association disorder: a problem where your child is unable to self-soothe and fall back to sleep on his own when he has brief normal arousals at night until certain conditions (the same as those present at time of sleep onset) are recreated for him.

Waking up too early in the morning:

Advanced sleep phase syndrome: another problem with the timing of sleep and wake, but in this case, your child has advanced his pattern, falling asleep and waking earlier than desired.

Many of these disorders and syndromes have been studied extensively by sleep specialists, but before we turn to describing their diagnosis and treatment, let's look at strategies for preventing sleep problems with improved, consistent sleep hygiene. In this case, a pound of prevention is worth a ton of cure.

Chapter 3

Sleep Hygiene

WHAT HAPPENS IN your home at night when it is time to put your child to bed? In many homes, where parents may be working long hours and may not have the support of extended family close by, the evening can be hectic. When you arrive at home after work, you contend with preparing dinner, tidying up, helping your children with homework, and, finally, trying to get them into bed. If this wasn't challenging enough, it is even harder to accomplish all these tasks when you, too, are exhausted.

The key to making the transition from daytime activities to nighttime sleep is to develop good sleep hygiene. Good sleep habits are fundamental for preventing your child from developing a sleep problem and the very first place to start if a problem already exists.

Did You Know?

Adult vs. Childhood Insomnia

When adults have insomnia or sleeplessness, they can educate themselves about improving sleep hygiene, understand the rationale, and make independent decisions about changing their sleep habits. Children, however, do not have the insight to change their sleep hygiene habits, so the responsibility for developing healthy sleep habits resides with the parents.

How Do I Develop Healthy Sleep Habits for My Children?

You can think of healthy sleep habits like other good habits in life. We teach our children at a young age to follow healthy habits so that they will become part of their daily or evening routines. For example, we may teach our children the habit of brushing their teeth every morning and evening, providing them with their own toothbrush and toothpaste, placing this in a designated place near the bathroom sink, and establishing a regular time for brushing. Children quickly learn these habits and follow a routine. After a while, there's no need to talk about the habit; it just gets done. Well, most of the time...

Good sleep hygiene is similar to good dental hygiene. There are habits you need to teach your children so they become routine. Even adults who have sleep problems could start by reviewing these healthy habits to see what they can improve in their own sleep hygiene or sleep health. You may be better prepared to help your child if you do so.

Behavioral Changes

First, you have to understand what needs to be changed and why, and then you need to introduce the changes slowly, along with rewards and consequences for your child's compliance to the new

case study: Vivian

Vivian's parents brought her to our office because she is always complaining of being tired, and in the last school term, her report card average dropped from a B to a C. Vivian is a 13-year-old girl with trouble settling to sleep at night due to problematic sleep habits. In her house, there is no routine or schedule. The family practices a relaxed, unstructured lifestyle. There are no rules about sleeping and waking.

When it comes to bedtime, Vivian goes to bed when she is tired. This can range from 9:00 p.m. to staying up as late as midnight. She gets to school each morning, but it's a big struggle. Often she misses breakfast, rushing to get to school on time. She always seems to be tired, even when she tries to catch up on her sleep on the weekends by sleeping until noon. Her parents asked us if we could help.

First, we helped her parents to identify Vivian's bad sleeping habits, and then we choose one habit at a time to change. We recommended establishing a bedtime routine. This could involve Vivian reading quietly in her bedroom for 30 minutes every night. At Vivian's age (13 years), she needs between 8.5 and 9.5 hours of sleep. If she has to wake up for school at 7:00 a.m., then she should be asleep between 9:30 and 10:30 p.m. They could start by setting her bedtime routine at 9:30 and lights out at 10:00, so that she can fall asleep by 10:30. After a week of this schedule, Vivian's bedtime routine could be moved 30 minutes earlier to 9:00 with lights out at 9:30, so that she is consistently falling asleep by 10:00 p.m.

Vivian's reward for cooperating with this new schedule should be something that she likes to do, rather than money or gifts. For a younger child, a reward could be a sticker chart, and if enough stickers are gained, a reward of special time with parents, a special activity, or time on the computer. For an older child or teenager, the reward could be similar, but chosen by the child/teenager and parents together, such as a movie night with friends. If Vivian does not cooperate, the consequences would be the removal of a privilege, such as computer time or a desired social outing or activity.

Using rewards and consequences, Vivian's parents gradually changed each problematic behavior and they were able to develop a regular routine and schedule for sleep and wake. Vivian is no longer overly tired during the day and her academic performance has improved.

routines. You might choose to make a sticker chart and decide with your child to adopt one new habit from the list below Then you can gradually work on each problematic behavior that you identify to promote better sleep hygiene in your child.

BAD SLEEP HABITS IDENTIFICATION WORKSHEET

In order to know where to start improving your child's sleep hygiene, you can work through the following list of bad sleep habits. Check off the behaviors your child exhibits and you permit. Then use the next worksheet to begin the process of gradually changing these problematic sleep habits.

❐ No bedtime routine

❐ No predictable bedtime

❐ No regular wake time

❐ Bedtime or wake time not consistent 7 days a week

❐ No expectations set by parents for consistency in schedules

❐ Large difference in sleep/wake times between school days and weekend days

❐ No regular mealtimes and often skips breakfast

❐ Eating heavy meals late at night

❐ Inadequate exercise or exercise late at night, close to bedtime

❐ Stimulating exercise, activity, discussion, computer or video games before bedtime instead of having quiet, relaxing, winding down time

❐ Sleeping in a bedroom that is noisy, light, or warm

❐ Child being in charge at bedtime (or anytime), demanding, for example, that only one parent can put her to bed

❐ Falling asleep out of the bedroom

❐ Falling asleep in bed with the television, radio, or music on

❐ Excessive caffeine intake, especially later in the afternoon and evening

❐ Not being exposed to sunlight in the morning

❐ Napping during the day, especially in the late afternoon (applies only to children beyond preschool)

❐ Use of nicotine, alcohol, or recreational drugs

BETTER SLEEP HYGIENE WORKSHEET

The following are some questions related to sleep hygiene. Fill in your answers to the following questions about sleep hygiene. Discussion of each question is then provided so you can take the first step to improving your child's sleep hygiene.

1. **Activities before bedtime:** What kind of activities does your child do between finishing supper and going to bed?

_____

_____

2. **Bedroom environment:** Is the bedroom she sleeps in quiet, comfortable, dark, and cool? Describe the bedroom atmosphere.

_____

_____

3. **Bedroom use:** What else is the bedroom used for? Does your child have a computer, television, MP3 player, telephone, or cell phone in the bedroom? How are these activities monitored at bedtime?

_____

_____

4. **Bedtime routine:** Do you have a bedtime routine? Is the bedtime routine short (under 30 minutes) and predictable? Does your child allow either parent to carry out the bedtime routine?

_____

_____

5. **Bedtime and wake time:** Does your child have a regular bedtime? Is this bedtime appropriate for your child's age, allowing time for sufficient sleep at night? Is it the same 7 days a week? Does your child have a regular wake time? Is it the same 7 days a week?

_____

_____

6. **Mealtimes:** During the day, are your child's meals regular? Are they regular 7 days a week?

_____

_____

7. **Caffeine:** Does you child eat or drink foods with caffeine? Take an inventory of the caffeine listed on food and drink nutritional facts labels.

_____

_____

8. **Exercise:** Does your child get regular exercise during the day? Does your child have any sport, dance, or other exercise activities in the evening after dinner? List these activities, their time, and their duration. (Remember that these evening activities are not problematic for all children. However, if your child has more trouble falling asleep after these stimulating evening activities, this should be noted here.)

_____

_____

9. **Sunlight:** Does your child get exposure to sunlight in the morning? List at what time and if the time is consistent 7 days per week.

_____

_____

10. **Naps:** Since the time that your child outgrew the habit of napping, has this practice resumed as an older child or teenager? List when this started and note the timing and duration of the naps.

_____

_____

11. **Nicotine, alcohol, and other substances:** Does your teenager smoke cigarettes (nicotine), drink alcohol, or use recreational drugs? This may be difficult to determine, but take the time to talk with your son or daughter.

_____

_____

Before Bedtime Activities

Good Evening Activities	Problematic Evening Activities
Relaxing activities, such as reading or listening to a story	Doing activities that cause excitement, stress, or anxiety, such as watching violence in a movie or computer game
Listening to music	Roughhousing with a family member
Playing a quiet game	Playing a competitive game or exercising vigorously 3 hours before bedtime
Taking a warm bath	Working on complicated homework or computer games within 1 hour of going to sleep
Talking in a calm way about the day	Discussing stressful situations or problems with your child just before it is time to fall asleep

Good Sleep Habits

Refer to your notes in the Better Sleep Hygiene Worksheet as we work through this corresponding list of good sleep habits.

Activities before Bedtime

Some activities help your child to sleep and some make it harder to fall asleep.

Bedroom Environment

Wherever your child sleeps, whether in his own room, in a shared room with a sibling, or in your room, he should have a space to sleep at night that is his own. This may be part of a shared bed or his own bed. Your child does not need to have his own room. In fact, many children prefer to sleep with a sibling. The important thing is that the bed (or the part of the bed, if he shares it with a sibling) has an adequate amount of space for sleeping.

> **Bedroom Qualities**
> - Quiet
> - Dark at night
>   (a night-light is fine)
> - Comfortable
> - Cool

Quiet

The bedroom must be quiet when your child is falling asleep. If you live in a noisy city, then you may need to use heavy blinds or curtains to create a quiet room. Your child should not fall asleep in a room with the television turned on or music playing. If your child shares a room with an older sibling, this may mean that the sibling has to do her homework outside of the bedroom at night. There should not be a lot of noise in the house from other parts of the home, from older siblings, or from television or music in other rooms.

Dark at Night

Light and darkness are major cues to tell our body when to be awake and when to fall asleep. Darkness triggers the production of a hormone called melatonin, which promotes sleep. For this reason, it is much healthier to fall asleep in a dark room. You may need to install blackout curtains to darken the room at night, though the bedroom does not have to be entirely dark. A night-light set at a low light will not affect sleep/wake rhythms. Full light triggers wakefulness, so it is equally important to have exposure to natural sunlight in the morning to help set the biological clock to 'wake up'.

Comfortable

Your child should have a comfortable mattress and feel safe in his bedroom. If your child has allergies, the room and pillows should be nonallergenic.

Cool

The bedroom should be at a comfortably cool temperature at night to promote sleep onset and maintain sleep. The temperature should be adjusted so that a lightly clothed adult would be comfortable. For younger infants and toddlers, you can ensure they have appropriate warm sleepers to stay comfortable if the covers are dislodged at night.

Bedroom Use

The bedroom should only be used for sleeping, especially if your child has difficulty falling asleep. Remove computers, telephones, radios, and televisions from your children's bedroom so that at bedtime, they can only use their bedroom to go to sleep. Some older children and teenagers who are anxious about falling asleep can also turn the clocks in the room toward the wall to prevent them from being overly focused on the time and their anxiety about falling asleep.

Bedtime Routine

Bedtime Routine Qualities
• Short
• Predictable
• Interchangeable

Try to establish a bedtime routine that is short, predictable, and consistent. The routine can change as the child grows, but even infants at a few months of age can benefit from a routine.

It is important for you and your partner to take turns with the bedtime routine. This doesn't have to be on any rigid schedule. Bedtime should be a happy, bonding time, and each parent should have the opportunity for this special activity. Your child should learn to allow either parent to share this bedtime routine. When your child allows each parent to participate in this activity, it becomes easier to transfer the routine to another family member or caregiver when parents are not available at bedtime.

Short

The bedtime routine should last for 15 to 30 minutes, and your child should learn that the end of the routine signifies time to go to sleep. The routine should be in the child's bedroom where it is quiet.

Predictable

The routine will change as your child grows, but it should remain predictable. When things are done in the exact same order (some children even like the exact same story and song for some time), this lets the child know that it is time to go to sleep and is comforted by its predictability each night.

Interchangeable

The routine should be able to be carried out by either parent or a caregiver. Your child should not be able to demand, for example, that Mommy always puts him to bed.

Bedtime and Wake Time

As much as possible (given the demands of daily life with its changing schedule), your child should have a bedtime and wake time that is the same 7 days a week. Bedtime will become later as your child grows up, but it should always be set to allow adequate sleep duration.

In older children and teenagers, who often have later bedtimes on the weekends, it is even more important to keep the wake time consistent.

Mealtimes

The timing of meals is important for keeping the 'biological clock' adjusted each day and maintaining a regular sleep-wake cycle. Food, like light, is a zeitgeber that helps us to set the internal clock and keep us on a 24-hour cycle. For this reason, your child should eat at the correct time of the day and avoid eating at the wrong time. This includes eating breakfast every morning at around the same time. Your child should avoid heavy meals late at night, which will disrupt sleep onset. A light carbohydrate snack, such as fruit or cheese and crackers, before bedtime, however, may help to induce sleep onset.

Sunlight

Your child should be exposed to natural light (sunlight) in the morning upon waking. Open the curtain in his bedroom in the morning to let in natural light. Sunlight and other sources of intense light are one of the strongest cues to tell us that it is time to wake up.

Caffeine

Caffeine is a stimulant that causes an alerting effect and can keep your child awake at night. If your child has caffeinated products in the afternoon or evening, the effect of the caffeine stays in the body for 3 to 5 hours, but it can have a longer-lasting effect, up to 12 hours. Be sure your child avoids caffeinated foods and beverages 6 hours before bedtime. Some soda drinks may have caffeine, so you need to check the caffeine content of food and drinks if you are not sure.

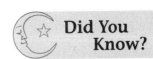

Did You Know?

Sunday Morning Wake-up
Some teenagers have difficulty getting up for school on Monday morning, especially if they are sleeping past noon on Sunday. To minimize disruption to their routine, they should wake up, especially on Sunday morning, no later than 1 hour after the time they wake up during the week.

Caffeine Content of Common Foods and Drinks

Product	Amount	Caffeine
Cola drinks (Coca-Cola or Pepsi)	8 oz	23–25 mg
Sweetened ice tea	8 oz	8–35 mg
Sunkist orange soda	8 oz	28 mg
Mountain Dew	8 oz	37 mg
Coffee	7 oz	80–135 mg
Decaffeinated coffee	7 oz	2–4 mg
Hot chocolate	7 oz	5 mg
Chocolate milk	8 oz	7–8 mg
Chocolate bar	45 g	30 mg
Energy drink	8 oz	80 mg

Did You Know?

Napping Benefits
Unfortunately, we do not have any studies on the benefits of napping in children who have outgrown the need for a nap. However, there have been studies on the benefits of napping in adults, which show that the effect of a daytime nap depends on the person's recent sleep pattern. If adults have a normal duration of sleep at night and have a nap of more than 30 minutes, the following day, they will have an improvement in alertness and performance following the nap.

Exercise

Regular exercise is not only important for your child's general health, but also for sleeping better at night. People who exercise find it easier to fall asleep at night and have deeper sleep. However, your child should not exercise vigorously at least 3 hours before bedtime. Exercising too close to bedtime may cause trouble in falling asleep because of excitement of the sport and increased body temperature. Body temperature typically begins to drop in the evening, which is associated with the timing of sleep onset.

Naps

While children generally outgrow their nap by the age of 5, everyone at every age finds that occasional napping is restful. It can be refreshing to have a regular, short nap in the early afternoon. The nap length should be more than 20 minutes or less than 90 minutes for maximum benefit. However, if your child has difficulty sleeping through the night or falling asleep, daytime sleep should be discouraged.

DAILY SLEEP HABITS GUIDE

Here are the principles of developing good sleep hygiene for a typical day in the life of your child. Consistency and regularity are the foundation of ongoing good sleep habits.

Morning

- Establish a consistent wake time: 7 days a week, including weekends and holidays.
- Eat breakfast at the same time every morning.
- Expose your child to direct sunlight in the morning, when possible.

Daytime

- Plan regular exercise for your child, such as biking, roller-blading, or hiking.
- Plan regular meals and snacks during the day.
- Limit your child's intake of caffeinated food or beverages (cola, chocolate, tea, coffee) and allow none of these for about 6 hours before bedtime. This is applicable to nicotine if your teenager smokes.
- If your child is napping, establish a regular nap schedule and wake him up from his afternoon nap by 4 p.m.

Early Evening

- Reserve this time for winding down, calm activities, and discussions.
- Discuss stressful situations and experiences during the day or now, not just before bedtime.
- Avoid vigorous exercise and sports from now until bedtime.
- Avoid your child's exposure to stimulating or violent television shows, computer programs, or video games.
- Don't allow your child to eat heavy meals.

Bedtime

- Your child can eat a light bedtime snack, if desired. Avoid excessive fluids.
- Do not allow your child to watch television in bed or have a television in his bedroom.
- If not already done, turn off your child's computer and cell phone.
- Consider giving your child a warm bath 60 to 90 minutes before sleep time. This may be helpful to some children and stimulating to others, so you need to determine if this is helpful.
- Provide a dark, quiet, comfortably cool room for your child.
- Let your child fall asleep on his own in his bedroom.

Nicotine and Alcohol

Teenagers generally know that smoking is bad for their health, but they may not be aware of the effects of nicotine on sleeping. Nicotine (in cigarettes and other tobacco products) acts as a stimulant and can make it more difficult to fall asleep at bedtime. Some teenagers think that alcohol helps them fall asleep, but it actually disrupts sleep, in addition to the other health dangers it can cause.

Sleep Hygiene through the Ages

Newborn (0–6 Months)

When your child is an infant, you will be caring for all his needs, including his sleep routine. While you can expect to be tired and sleep deprived during this time, there's no need for your baby to be. Although his sleep pattern may wear you out, when your newborn has grown into a teenager who is independent and wants to sleep until noon, you may reflect longingly on those early days when he was a baby and waking you through the night.

NEWBORN SLEEP ROUTINE

To establish and maintain good sleep habits for your baby:

- Provide a safe sleep environment.

- Put your baby to sleep on her back.

- Some babies can fall asleep on their own. Others need to be nurtured and helped to fall asleep by feeding, rocking, and cuddling.

- Look for the signs that your baby is getting sleepy (usually within 2 hours after the last feeding) and help him fall asleep when you see these signs.

- Help your baby to learn the difference between day and night by waking him in the morning, playing with him during the day more than in the evening, and putting him to bed at night. Some babies get their days and nights mixed up.

- Provide a dark room at night and natural light during the day. Have your supplies close at hand to change diapers and use a night-light to decrease stimulation at night. During the day, let natural light into the room when your baby is napping.

- Get as much sleep for yourself as possible.

After several months of following a routine, you will notice the changes in your baby's sleep behavior. Your child will begin to sleep for longer periods, more so at night. Your baby will be more wakeful during the day. Some babies will naturally start to sleep through the night, but if your baby does not do this, there are techniques to encourage longer sleep periods. These techniques, called behavior management, have been shown in research studies to be effective.

Q. **How often should my baby wake at night?**

A. Frequent waking at night in babies is one of the most frequent sleep concerns of parents. When your infant is a newborn, you can expect to be woken frequently at night (from two to five times) to feed and change him. This is part of the normal newborn sleep pattern.

Q. **What can I do to teach my baby to sleep longer periods at night?**

A. Although some babies can settle on their own, even as newborns, other need to be nurtured to sleep. For the first few months of life, you should help your infant to fall asleep by rocking, cuddling, nursing, and bottle-feeding, or any other soothing, nurturing technique. You cannot 'spoil' your baby by providing this comfort, despite what your well-intentioned relatives or friends may tell you. Your baby needs this contact while falling asleep. Babies cannot always soothe themselves independently.

As your child develops more mature sleep patterns by 3 to 4 months of age, you can start to put your baby to bed drowsy but awake. You can still stay with him while he is falling asleep, feeding, rocking, or patting him in his crib, but you can start to decrease the soothing activities that he needed for the first few months of life. As long as your baby is thriving, by the time he is 6 months of age, you can start to decrease his nighttime feeding if you want to encourage longer sleep periods at night, and he will gradually eat more during the day to make up for the changes.

Q. **My baby has her days and nights mixed up. How do I reverse her schedule?**

A. A newborn up to 3 months of age has not developed a circadian rhythm and wakes and sleeps according to her need to drink or her need for comfort, rather than to a day/night schedule. Even with a young baby, you can decrease the stimulation that you provide when she wakes at night and increase your play with her during the day. When your baby wakes at night, you should take care of her needs, but do this calmly and quietly. You should feed and change her, but do this in a dimly lit room, without turning on music or talking to her loudly. This lack of stimulation will encourage her to return to sleep. However, during the day, you can be more playful when your baby wakes to eat, turning on the lights, singing to her, and talking to her. These activities will encourage her to stay awake longer between feedings than during the night. Using these methods, she will gradually reverse her schedule and sleep longer at night and stay awake longer during the day. You should expect this change to take place by 6 months of age.

Younger Infant (4 to 6 Months)

After 4 to 6 months of your sleep being disrupted, you may become mildly to severely sleep deprived. This can affect your ability to cope. The amount of sleep deprivation you experience will depend on many factors relating to your baby's sleep, your own need for sleep, your general medical health, and your support at home. You may be able to obtain some sleep during the day when your baby sleeps. But the most important thing you can do to improve your sleep is to establish a sleep routine for your child to give both of you more rest.

Q. **What does 'sleeping through the night' mean?**

A. Prominent pediatric sleep researchers studying infant wake and sleep patterns extensively define 'sleeping through the night' as sleeping from midnight until 5:00 a.m. They have found that, although parents may report that their infant sleeps through the night, when you videotape infants sleeping, you see the brief arousals that are a normal part of sleep. These infants are able to soothe themselves easily back to sleep without 'signaling' the need for parental intervention. In considering whether you need to improve your infant's sleep routine, it would be a good goal for a 6-month-old infant to be sleeping without signaling you upon his brief nocturnal arousals for 6 or more hours, although research studies have shown that 30% of babies at this age do not sleep for at least 6 hours at night. As your infant gets older, your expectation for longer sleep periods at night would also lengthen.

YOUNGER INFANT (4 TO 6 MONTHS) SLEEP ROUTINE

To establish and maintain good sleep habits for your young infant:

- Establish a routine, even if it is very short (5 minutes to start), that will help teach your baby that something special happens just before bedtime. This could be as simple as singing the same lullaby or reading the same simple story at bedtime.

- Keep the routine consistent, putting your baby to bed in the same room. For an infant, consistency would mean that, whenever possible, your baby is in his own crib at home or daycare for naps and bedtime. Depending on your family life, work, and household responsibilities, you may find yourself letting your baby sleep in the car or the stroller frequently. This is not a problem for all babies. However, when possible, you should allow your baby to start her nap at similar times during the day, have a similar bedtime, and sleep in her own crib.

- Stop feeding your baby when he is drowsy but full. Instead of nursing or feeding him until he is fast asleep, put him in the crib (on his back) drowsy and let him learn to fall asleep without drinking at the same time. If he is bottle-feeding, don't give him his bottle when you place him in the crib as he falls asleep.

- Try using a transitional object, such as a blanket or stuffed animal, that lets your child know it is bedtime. For a young infant, this can be sleeping with the same blanket in the crib. For a toddler or older child, this may be a soft stuffed animal or blanket.

- Give your child cues or signs that lets him know there is a difference between night and day. You want to help your baby to learn that night is for sleeping and day is for being awake. Although he doesn't know this intuitively, he will learn by recognizing that you interact with him differently at night than during the day. Babies enjoy all the positive attention and cuddling that you provide. If you start to decrease (not stop) this positive interaction at night when your baby wakes up, he will slowly adjust to waking for shorter times at night and anticipate being awake in the daytime for your concentrated attention.

- Slowly decrease the amount of stimulation (light, noise, cuddling) you give your baby when he wakes during the night and increase the playful times you have with him during the day.

- When you are feeding your infant or changing his diapers during night wakings, keep the room light dim (just enough light to care safely for your baby) and speak quietly.

Q. **How can I get my baby to sleep through the night? Should I just let him 'cry it out'?**

A. You may have been advised to just let your baby 'cry it out' and not respond to him at night. This method of improving your baby's sleep is not recommended. There is a concern about potential harm caused by being nonresponsive to your infant. Infants signal their needs by crying – this is your baby's way of communicating with you. If you do not respond at all when she cries, you won't know the cause of the crying, and your baby may receive the message that her caregiver cannot be relied on for meeting her needs. You will learn methods to teach your baby to sleep through the night in the following chapters.

Older Infant (6 to 12 months)

At this age, your baby will go for longer periods between feedings. A healthy 6-month-old, full-term baby can learn to sleep for longer periods at night. By 9 months of age, 70% to 80% of babies will sleep through the night (at least 6 hours at a time).

This is a good time to establish healthy sleep habits by helping your child learn to sleep for longer periods at night without needing to nurse or bottle-feed, or to require parental intervention to return to sleep at times of brief nocturnal arousals.

Q. **Why do some infants wake frequently at night?**

A. At this age, the most common sleep problem is frequent waking at night. In some families, this is not a problem if the mother or caregiver is willing to wake up frequently with the baby and feed him through the night. If you prefer to do this, and your baby is thriving, go ahead. This pattern can resolve on its own in some babies who learn naturally to sleep through the night. In other babies, where the mother or caregiver wants to increase nighttime sleep, some sleep training is needed.

Your baby may awake and cry out because he is hungry and thirsty. Most babies who wake frequently at night fall asleep easily after being breast-fed or bottle-fed. However once asleep, they may wake up many times at night and will only go back to sleep once they are fed again. This becomes a hard problem to solve because the more they eat, the thirstier and hungrier they are at night. Frequent feeding becomes a habit. In addition, frequent fluids may cause your baby to urinate often and so he may waken due to a wet diaper.

(continued at right...)

OLDER INFANT (6–12 MONTHS) SLEEP ROUTINE

To establish and maintain good sleep habits for your older infant:

- Provide a safe sleep environment. Continue to have your baby sleep in his crib for the first year of life. Toward the end of the first year, when your baby may be standing in the crib, you should remove the side bumpers (if you have been using them) and make sure the crib mattress is at the lowest setting. It is recommended not to use bumper pads even with infants, but if you have them in the bed, you should remove them at this stage.

- Continue with the regular bedtime routine at naps and nighttime. Change the routine as your baby develops, adding a story at bedtime, for example.

- Put your baby in bed awake and leave the room, allowing her to fall asleep on her own.

- Look for the signs your baby is sleepy and put her to bed at these times. Avoid putting her in bed when she is not sleepy as this will increase the time she is unhappy and unable to fall asleep.

- Allow your baby to decrease his naps from three to four a day in infancy to two naps (one in the morning and the other in early afternoon) by the end of the first year.

- Promote longer sleep periods by avoiding naps in the late afternoon. During the days, naps should be at regular times for a consistent duration.

A. *(...continued)*

If you want to lengthen your baby's sleep at night, you can change this pattern of frequent feeding. A healthy 6-month-old baby can learn to sleep long periods at night without food. But if you suddenly stop feeding your baby and expect her to learn to sleep through the night, she will still wake up because she is both thirsty and hungry. She is used to having a certain amount of calories and fluid during the night, and needs to change this habit gradually. Watering down your baby's milk or replacing milk with water (if he is being bottle-fed) is likewise not effective.

Research studies support the value of using behavioral techniques to improve sleep in infants. Your baby can learn to sleep through the habit of frequent feeding if you decrease the nighttime feedings slowly so that her hunger will be satisfied during the day, instead of during the night. Over time, she will consume the same amount of calories and fluid in a 24-hour period, but can learn to do this during daytime hours, from 6:00 a.m. to 10:00 p.m. or midnight.

Q. My baby is teething and this is disrupting her sleep. What should I do?

A. Babies will begin to have teeth erupt between 5 and 8 months of life. Although your baby may have some pain from this, you will know when the pain is at its worst because just before a tooth erupts, the gums will be red and slightly swollen. On these days, her sleep may be disrupted. However, teething will not be a cause of ongoing sleep problems.

Toddlers and Preschool Children

The toddler years are full of fun during the day, but can be challenging at night. When your child moves from his crib to a bed and gains new independence in his motor skills, this can provide new ways to resist staying in bed and falling asleep at night. This is also the time, if your child has been sleeping in his crib in your room, to move him to his own or shared bedroom with a sibling. This may also be the time when the bedtime routine becomes sporadic because you are working outside of the home and conflicted between your desire to get your child to bed or to spend more time together at night.

TODDLER AND PRESCHOOL CHILD SLEEP ROUTINE

To establish and maintain good sleep habits for your toddler:

- Provide a safe, comfortable quiet, dimly lit, slightly cool bedroom environment. Try to have your child nap and sleep in his bed in this room.

- Maintain a consistent schedule for naps and bedtime with a predictable, short naptime and bedtime routine.

- Leave your child in his bed in the room while he is awake and let him learn to fall asleep alone.

- Try to keep this routine as much as possible 7 days a week, with a predictable time for sleep and waking.

- Encourage the use of a transitional object if your child is having trouble being alone or separating himself from you.

- Put your child to bed when he is showing signs of sleepiness.

- Help him to transition from a crib to a bed, when he is able to get out of the crib independently.

Q. My child is not sleepy enough to need two naps, but if I let him have his morning nap and miss the afternoon one, he is cranky in the afternoon and falls asleep too early at night. How do I get him to have enough sleep with one nap in the day?

A. You can help your child transition from two naps to one nap. Instead of letting him miss his afternoon nap, let him miss the morning nap. Keep the afternoon nap, but move it earlier in the day. Initially, you can move his whole schedule earlier, letting him have an earlier lunch, start his nap before noon, and have an earlier bedtime. Over time, you can gradually move his schedule a little later – for example, you can delay his lunch, his nap time, and his bedtime by 15 minutes each week for 3 to 6 weeks until he is able to stay awake for the whole morning and have one nap in the afternoon.

School-Age Children (6 to 12 Years)

Parents of children between the ages of 6 and 12 often have concerns about their child's sleep. Up to one-quarter of children at this age will continue to have difficulty falling asleep at night. In addition, approximately 30% of children in this age group have problems with bed-wetting, sleepwalking, sleep talking, or nighttime fears. These problems are described in the following chapters. Whether your school-age child has sleep problems or not, the following routines are helpful to establish good sleep hygiene at this age.

SCHOOL-AGE CHILD SLEEP ROUTINE

To establish and maintain good sleep habits for your school-age child:

- Provide an appropriate sleep environment with a transitional object, if accepted. Remove television, computer, telephone, and music from the bedroom if they are interfering with sleep onset or continuity.

- Maintain a consistent, regular bedtime 7 days a week (if possible). The time should be appropriate for your child's age.

- Maintain a consistent wake time 7 days a week.

- Establish a quiet time before bedtime. Avoid vigorous activity or stimulating games for 1 to 2 hours before bedtime.

- Avoid caffeinated foods and beverages from mid-afternoon onward.

- Monitor exposure to violent or inappropriate media.

- Allow your child to fall asleep alone, without either parent present.

Adolescents

In the teenage years, sleep and wake issues can be challenging for you and for your teen. As in other areas of your teenager's life, you may not have the same authority or control as in previous years. The advice your teenager gets from his friends, teachers, or even the Internet may be of greater importance than information parents offer.

However, you can assure your teenager that there have been scientific studies done on sleep during the teenage years that you can share with him. If your teenager is experiencing problems due to inadequate or irregular sleep, share this book with him and discuss together how you can work to resolve his sleeping difficulties.

ADOLESCENT SLEEP ROUTINE

To establish and maintain good sleep habits for your adolescent:

- Curtail participation in stimulating activities close to bedtime – playing active sports, watching stimulating television and videos.

- Encourage using the bed for sleeping, not for watching television, playing on a portable computer, talking on the phone.

- Discourage use of caffeine, nicotine, and other drugs (prescription or otherwise) to stay awake in the afternoon and evening.

- Monitor the bedroom environment to ensure it is not too light, too hot, too cold, or too noisy so that it does not interfere with sleep onset.

- Help your teenager to maintain a consistent bedtime and wake time, 7 days a week (if possible).

Q. Can my teenager's problem falling asleep be something more serious than poor sleep hygiene?

A. You need to understand what is the problem preventing your child from falling asleep and causing sleep onset insomnia. If the problem goes beyond poor sleep hygiene as the cause of inadequate sleep, it may be delayed sleep phase syndrome, a problem that can often be successfully treated by following the steps in this book. If you suspect that the problem is related to a medical condition, mood disorder, or other serious problem, your child may need to see his health-care provider. Another cause of insomnia, which can be first noticed in the teenage years, is primary insomnia. This is a problem that can start even in childhood and cause chronically poor sleep. If your teenager has adequate sleep hygiene and does not have a delayed sleep phase, signs of depression, or other medical or psychiatric problems, he may have primary insomnia. This type of insomnia can also be treated successfully.

Chapter 4

Sleep Safety

I F YOU ARE A new parent or parent-to-be, you are probably making many plans for your baby, including where your child will sleep. Will your baby sleep on her own in her own room and in her own crib? Will she sleep with a sibling in the same room, or will she sleep in your room? If she sleeps in your room, will she sleep with you in bed or in her own bassinet or crib? Your decisions will be influenced by your cultural background and experience, as well as discussions with your physician, family, and friends.

There are many different sleeping arrangements that are acceptable. In many cultures, children sleep with their parents or siblings, either in the same bed or in the same room. Pediatric associations in the United States and Canada recommend that the best place for your baby to sleep is definitely in the same room as you during the first 6 months, but in his own crib. In addition, it is recommended that your baby sleep in his own crib for the first year of life.

Despite this recommendation, controversy arises among some sleep and breast-feeding experts whether you should co-sleep with your baby (bed-sharing). Bed-sharing has been shown to increase slightly the risk of sudden infant death syndrome (SIDS). A similar concern has recently been raised by some experts over the recommendation of the American Academy of Pediatrics to use pacifiers in infants in an attempt to decrease the risk of SIDS. There is also some controversy about co-sleeping or bed-sharing with a toddler or child. While common in many cultures, this practice may affect your child's sleep pattern adversely, especially if the bed-sharing is reactive in the attempt to soothe a chronically sleepless child.

Although there is no single correct sleeping arrangement, you should be aware of the benefits and risks of these various arrangements so that you can make an informed decision for your family, along with knowledge about risk factors for SIDS.

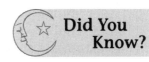

Did You Know?

Room-Sharing Safety
It is recommended that your baby sleep in your bedroom until the age of 6 months. Research studies show that when a committed caregiver sleeps in the same room, but not in the same bed with an infant, the chance of the infant dying from SIDS is reduced by 50%. In these studies, the committed caregiver is usually the mother, but can be the father.

What is SIDS?

Sudden infant death syndrome (SIDS) describes the sudden and unexpected death of an apparently healthy baby under 1 year of age. The baby's death is assumed to be from SIDS if, despite a thorough investigation, which includes a complete autopsy, examination of the death scene, and review of the clinical history, there is no explanation for the child's death. There are several theories about the cause of SIDS, including the possibility that the baby who dies from SIDS has a deficiency in his ability to arouse from deep sleep.

SIDS FACTS

- Although SIDS can occur up to 1 year of age, it is most likely to happen between the ages of 2 and 4 months.

- The rate of SIDS has decreased by more than 50% in both Canada and the United States between 1990 and 2002. In Canada, the rate has fallen from 0.8 per 1000 live babies born in 1990 to 0.3 per 1000 live babies born in 2002. The rate of SIDS in the United States has fallen from 1.3 to 0.6 per 1000 live babies born from 1990 to 2002.

- The decrease in SIDS is due to increased public awareness that babies should sleep on their backs. When the American public received education about this in the Back to Sleep campaign between 1992 and 2002, surveys showed that the number of babies who slept on their tummies fell from 70% to 11.3% and the incidence of SIDS fell by 50% from 1.2 babies for every 1000 live births in 1992 to 0.57 babies for each 1000 live births in 2002.

Did You Know?

Tummy vs. Back Sleep
Putting your baby to sleep on his tummy is associated with an increased risk of SIDS, whether you are co-sleeping or not, but may be recommended by your doctor in special circumstances. When babies sleep on their backs, they cry more often and arouse more often because they do not sleep as deeply. However, a lighter sleep may be protective against SIDS.

Pre-Natal SIDS Prevention

Even before your baby is born, you can reduce the risk of SIDS by:
- Getting regular prenatal care to help reduce the risk of having a premature baby, which is a risk factor for SIDS.

- Not smoking or using illicit drugs during your pregnancy, which is a risk factor for SIDS.

- Spacing your pregnancies. If you wait at least 1 year between the birth of your baby and your next pregnancy, this will reduce the risk of SIDS.

Co-Sleeping with an Infant

Co-sleeping can include several different arrangements, each with their own merits. Discuss the benefits and risks of your chosen sleeping arrangement with your baby's doctor. If you decide to bed-share, then you need to do so in the safest way possible. Weigh the benefits and risks carefully.

case study: **Lauren and Kyle**

Lauren and Kyle are expecting their first child. Lauren is in her third trimester. They came to our clinic to discuss issues about caring for their newborn, including breast-feeding and co-sleeping. Lauren is hoping to breast-feed her baby. She has researched the pros and cons of breast-feeding and bottle-feeding, and feels that breast-feeding is the healthiest option. However, Lauren and Kyle are confused about whether it is safe or not to co-sleep with the baby in their bed. They want to know what the risks and benefits are of this arrangement.

We reinforced Lauren's decision to breast-feed as the best way to feed her baby. Breast-feeding has many benefits, both for mothers and babies. We also presented Lauren and Kyle with some of the key information about keeping their baby safe while sleeping, especially what the American and Canadian pediatric societies recommend, based on the evidence about SIDS. We advised them to sleep in the same room as their baby, with the baby in a separate sleeping space but close-by, in a crib or bassinet.

Room-Sharing with Parents

In this type of co-sleeping arrangement, your baby sleeps in his own crib or bassinet in the same room with you. The American Academy of Pediatrics and the Canadian Paediatric Society both recommend this sleeping arrangement, for several reasons.

Room-Sharing Benefits

- If your baby sleeps in your bedroom in his own crib close to your bed, you will be able to easily respond to his needs during the night.
- This sleeping arrangement is one factor associated with a decreased risk of SIDS.

Bed-sharing with Parents

You and your baby, with or without your partner, share an adult bed and sleep together on the same sleeping surface. Bed-sharing with parents is the most common sleeping arrangement worldwide and families may choose to bed-share because of cultural, parenting, or family beliefs. Some experts advocate bed-sharing if done in a 'safe way' for several reasons. Bed-sharing will encourage ease of breast-feeding, which has important benefits not only for your baby, but also for you. But there are also risks to be considered, including overheating and overlying.

Bed-Sharing Benefits

- Bed-sharing may improve breast-feeding due to the convenience of sleeping next to your baby.
- Babies who breast-feed and bed-share have more arousals, as do their mothers. When your child wakes, you will be more likely to wake also and able to respond easily to his needs.
- If you are breast-feeding your baby in bed and fall asleep, this is a safer place for your baby than if you fall asleep while feeding him in a chair or sofa.

Bed-Sharing Risks

- Infants who bed-share are at increased risk of SIDS, due to several factor. Although the exact mechanism of SIDS is not known, these factors may put the child at risk of overlying, overheating, or lack of arousal.
- If more than one parent is in the bed.
- If the infant is sleeping on an adult bed, in an armchair, or on a sofa.
- If a mother is obese.
- If a parent is on sedating medication, under the influence of alcohol or drugs, or extremely fatigued.
- The baby may become overheated because of a warm room or too many bedclothes.
- If a bed has soft bedding, pillows, and comforters, which may cover your baby's head and face.
- An unsafe bed. There are safety standards applied to the construction of cribs, crib mattresses, and bassinets for babies, but there are no safety standards for adult beds in which babies are sleeping.
- If a parent smokes in the room or in bed. Exposure to environmental tobacco smoke at any time is a risk factor for SIDS, not only if the mother smokes during pregnancy, but also if your baby once born is exposed to smoke from anyone in the home. This tobacco smoke-related risk increases if you bed-share.

Co-Sleeping without Bed-Sharing

In this case, you and your baby sleep beside each other at the same level, but not on the same sleeping surface. The benefit and risks of this arrangement are not well understood; this sleeping arrangement is less common in most developed countries.

Did You Know?

Benefits and Risks
Some families will choose a bed-sharing sleeping arrangement even though they are aware of the recommendations against it because of the benefits, recognizing the actual increased risk of SIDS, although real, is small.

Bed-Sharing with Others, Not Parents

Your baby shares a bed or a room with someone other than you or your partner. Experts agree that if your baby is sharing a bed, it should not be with anyone other than his parent or usual caregiver. This arrangement does not have any benefit to the safety of your baby. This arrangement does not decrease the risk of SIDS because a person who is not the parent or usual caregiver of your baby will be much less likely to rouse easily or be responsive to your baby's needs during sleep.

PEDIATRIC ASSOCIATION GUIDELINES

The Canadian Paediatric Society (2004) and the American Academy of Pediatrics (2005) have published similar guidelines for creating a safe sleeping environment for your baby and decreasing the risk of SIDS:

- For the first year of your baby's life, the safest place to sleep is in his own crib, on his back. This should be the way you place your baby in the crib to sleep for naps and at bedtime.

- The crib, bassinet, or cradle must meet the safety standards of the country in which you live.

- For the first 6 months, your baby should sleep in the parents' bedroom in his own crib, but close to you.

- When your baby can turn over on his own, there's no need to force your baby into the back sleep position. Foam wedges or towel rolls to keep babies on their side should not be used.

- Your baby should sleep on a firm surface, such as a firm crib mattress, covered by a sheet. Infants should never sleep on pillows, air mattresses, waterbeds, cushions, soft materials, or loose bedding. Keep soft objects, such as stuffed toys, away from the infant's sleeping environment. Plastics, including the manufacturer's mattress wrapping, should be removed from the mattress.

- The sleeping environment for infants should be free of quilts, comforters, bumper pads, pillows, and pillow-like items.

- Even when you are traveling, your baby must have a safe place to sleep. Car seats and infant carriers are not to be used to replace the crib for your baby's sleeptime.

- A baby should sleep in a room that is quiet, dark, and slightly cool. The room temperature should be comfortable for a lightly clothed adult. If the room temperature is comfortable for you, it should be right for your baby too.

- Keep your baby away from cigarette smoke. Babies whose mothers smoked during pregnancy and babies who continue to be exposed to smoke after birth are at an increased risk of SIDS.

- Never nap or sleep with your baby or let your baby sleep alone on a couch, sofa, or armchair.

- Consider dressing your baby in sleepers so that you don't need a blanket to cover her.

- If using a blanket, put your baby with his feet at the foot of the crib. Tuck a thin blanket around the crib mattress, reaching only as far as the baby's chest.

- Make sure your baby's head remains uncovered during sleep.

- Make sure everyone who cares for your baby knows the recommendations for safe sleeping.

- Your baby should not share a bed with other siblings or family members.

- It is acceptable to bring your baby into the bed to be breast-fed, and then he should be placed back into his crib or bassinet before you fall back asleep.

- In order to prevent your baby from having a flattened back of head (called positional plagiocephaly) from sleeping on his back, allow him time during the day when he is awake to play on his tummy.

- Because babies tend to turn their head toward the bedroom door to see who is coming and going, periodically alternate the direction your child is sleeping so that she will spend time looking both ways.

Room-Sharing with Others, Not Parent

Your baby may share a room with siblings or another family member. This may be your choice or due to the space available in your home. Sharing a room with others who are not the parents or usual caregiver has not been associated with a decreased risk of SIDS. This means that you wouldn't expect a family member, sibling, or grandparent to be as aware of your infant during sleep as you would be. There is no particular benefit with regards to decreasing the risk of SIDS to this sleeping arrangement for your baby; however, it may be the chosen arrangement in your family for other reasons.

Pacifiers and SIDS

The use of pacifiers has been associated with a reduced risk of SIDS. While pacifiers are often used to soothe a child to sleep, they can also disrupt his sleep — your baby gets used to falling asleep with one and you have to keep replacing it at night when he wakens to help him fall back to sleep. There are several theories as to how a pacifier may be associated with a reduced risk of SIDS; however, the exact reason for this is not known.

Based on the evidence from some studies, the American Academy of Pediatrics (AAP) in 2005 has issued a policy statement recommending the use of pacifiers to reduce the risk of SIDS in infants. In breast-fed babies, it is recommended to delay the introduction of the pacifier until 1 month of age after nursing is well established.

AMERICAN ACADEMY OF PEDIATRICS RECOMMENDATION ON PACIFIERS

The exact wording of the recommendation of the American Academy of Pediatrics (AAP) from their policy statement published in the journal *Pediatrics* in November 2005 is as follows:

"Consider offering a pacifier at naptime and bedtime. Although the mechanism is not known, the reduced risk of SIDS associated with pacifier use during sleep is compelling, and, on the other hand, the evidence that pacifier use inhibits breast-feeding or causes later dental complications is not. Until evidence dictates otherwise, the task force [of experts who reviewed this new research] recommends the use of a pacifier throughout the first year of life according to the following procedures:

- The pacifier should be used when placing the infant down for sleep and should not be reinserted once the infant falls asleep. If the infant refuses the pacifier, he should not be forced to take it.

- Pacifiers should not be coated in any sweet solution.

- Pacifiers should be cleaned often and replaced regularly.

- For breast-fed infants, delay pacifier introduction until 1 month of age to ensure that breast-feeding is firmly established."

In the same way that a baby who sleeps on his back will rouse more easily, a baby with a pacifier may also sleep less deeply. There are other reasons postulated for this association between pacifiers and a reduced risk of SIDS. If your baby uses a pacifier, he is more likely to sleep on his back. In the research examining this association, mothers who gave their babies pacifiers were less likely to smoke, so it may have been the lack of smoke in the environment, rather than the use of the pacifier, that decreased the incidence of SIDS.

Pacifier Controversy

There are other experts who argue that the evidence for recommending pacifier use to decrease the risk of SIDS is flawed, and that pacifiers have other potential adverse consequences for your baby's sleep.

- The research only shows that there is an association between pacifier use and a decrease in SIDS, not that using a pacifier will prevent a baby from dying from SIDS.

- The experts have made recommendations regarding pacifier use based on studies that look backward and rely on parent's memory about the past use of pacifiers.

- One of the theories about preventing SIDS by using a pacifier is that your baby will not sleep as deeply. Therefore, it is possible (but not yet studied) that the risk of SIDS will be decreased, but there may be consequences to growth and development that we do not know at this time from this effect.

- Pacifier use may interfere with breast-feeding. It is known that there is an association between pacifier use and breast-feeding duration, but not that pacifier use causes mothers to stop breast-feeding. The studies used to make the recommendation to use a pacifier did not differentiate between babies who were breast-fed and those who were not, so it is not known what is the role of pacifier use in a breast-fed baby for preventing SIDS.

- Pacifiers can be a source of germs if not properly cleansed. This problem can be dealt with by ensuring that your baby's pacifier is properly cleansed.

- Using a pacifier may cause sleep onset association problems, which can lead to more arousals at night and disruptive sleep. This may lead to more long-lasting sleep problems.

Did You Know?

Deep to Lighter Sleep
Pacifiers, like having a baby sleep on his back, will cause a baby to sleep less deeply. We do not know at this time if changing deep to lighter sleep will be detrimental for your baby since we all, especially as babies, need deep sleep for its restorative benefits.

Recommendations

Because research on the use of pacifiers is ongoing and controversial, we recommend that you discuss this issue with your doctor to ensure that you are making a decision based on the most current studies.

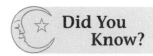

Did You Know?

Co-Sleeping with a Toddler or Older Child

After the first year of life, the risk of SIDS is no longer a reason for your toddler to sleep solitary in his own bed. If you want to co-sleep with your toddler, it is now safe, though you may prefer for your baby to continue sleeping solitary and not share the 'family bed'. Once again, you need to weigh the benefits and risks of these different sleeping arrangements.

Benefits and Risks

Co-sleeping with your toddler or older child is the norm for families in many cultures around the world. However, there are no studies yet comparing the benefits or risks for children when they sleep in the parental bed as a custom or when they are brought into the parents' bed because they have a sleep problem.

Potential Conflicts
Co-sleeping to resolve problems can cause potential conflicts both during the day and at bedtime between parents, between parent and child, and between the identified problem sleeper in the family and other siblings, which will affect the success of this method of sleeping.

case study: Jenny

Jenny is 4 years old. Both her parents work out of the home, but Jenny goes happily to nursery school in the morning and day care in the afternoon. Since the age of 2, when she began to climb out of her crib, she has slept with her parents in their bed. She sleeps quietly and her parents do not have any problems with this sleeping arrangement. In fact, due to their busy work schedule, they enjoy the family time together at bedtime and even during the night.

This may sound like a happy arrangement, but the 'family bed' can become problematic when the family grows. Jenny's mother is expecting a baby soon, and she is worried that the bed will not be big enough for the entire family. Now that Jenny has had 4 years of time alone with her parents, including sleeping with them for 2 years, her parents are worried about how she will adjust to having a new sibling in the bed and to the disruption to her time alone at night with her parents. In Jenny's case, her parents may choose to continue to sleep as a family or to move Jenny into her own room and bed gradually.

Reactive Co-Sleeping

In a family that co-sleeps in a reactive way, the parents prefer the child to sleep independently, either separately in her own room or with a sibling. Due to a sleep disturbance (for example, difficulty falling asleep or sleeping through the night), the parent brings the child into the parental bed to try to resolve the sleep problem.

case study: Maxine

Maxine's parents, Maria and Joe, came to our clinic because they were having difficulty getting Maxine to sleep at night. Maxine is 5 years old, healthy and energetic, but demanding. For the past 6 months. Maria and Joe have been trying different ways to get Maxine to sleep in her own room. These have included a sticker chart to reward her for cooperating, explaining to her why she must go to sleep at night, and disciplining her for not cooperating. After a few days of each method, Maria and Joe are so tired at night that they just give in, and, eventually, they fall back to the same routine of having Maxine in bed with them.

They have a double bed, but because Maxine is so restless at night, the three of them cannot fit into it comfortably. Joe ends up every night in Maxine's room, and Maxine and Maria sleep together. Maria is also tired of having to lie down with Maxine to fall asleep. Maria would really like to have some time in the evening with her husband and be able to sleep with him in their bed.

After we explored this problem with Maria and Joe, they realized that Maxine had to learn to fall asleep alone in her own room so that she would be able to do this during the night when she naturally woke. Learning to fall asleep in her own room at bedtime would enable her to fall back to sleep in her own room during the night. We provided Maria and Joe with several techniques for achieving this goal, explaining that they needed to be consistent and persistent. After all, Maxine had developed her sleep difficulties over 5 years, and it would take more than a few days to change them. Within 1 month, Maxine's sleep was much improved. She was able to fall asleep and stay asleep in her own room, and for the first time in 5 years, Maria and Joe had time alone at night together.

REASONS FOR CO-SLEEPING WITH YOUR TODDLER AND CHILD

Reasons to choose co-sleeping:

- Your cultural beliefs are that a child should not be alone at night.

- Your child or family has undergone a recent stressful event, move, illness, or burglary, for example, and this is a temporary family choice.

- You do not have adequate rooms or beds in your home for everyone to have a separate space at night.

Reasons to avoid co-sleeping:

- You are too tired at night to try any other method of sleeping arrangement to get your child to sleep independently, although this would not be your desired choice.

- This the only way that you can get your child to fall asleep and sleep through the night.

- You or your partner are working late and you just want more time in the presence of your child, regardless of whether you are awake or asleep.

- You fall asleep at night in your child's bed or with him in your bed, and then you are too tired to move or move him.

- This is the only way that you and the rest of your family get some sleep at night.

- You or your partner prefers the company of your child in bed to avoid marital communication and intimacy.

Changing Co-Sleeping Behavior

Co-sleeping with your toddler or child can be part of your family's chosen routine or it can be problematic. If everyone is happy with this arrangement, there can be benefits to your child and to the family. However, when you would prefer not to co-sleep and are only doing this because there is no other way to get your child to sleep at night, then you should try to resolve the problem. You can do this by following the advice in Part 3 (Step-by-Step Guide to Better Sleep) of this book about how to change the problematic pattern and help your children learn to sleep through the night either with a sibling or on their own.

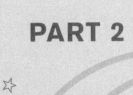

PART 2

Sleep Disorders

CHAPTER 1 Signs and Symptoms of Sleep Disorders 68

CHAPTER 2 Treatment of Sleep Disorders 78

Chapter 1

Signs and Symptoms of Sleep Disorders

A SLEEP DISTURBANCE CAN refer to many problems that interfere with adequate sleep (in quality or quantity) or with normal waking behavior. Most, but not all, sleep disturbances cause problems during the day, including daytime fatigue, difficult behavior, poor attention, memory problems, or learning difficulties for your child. Some sleep disorders, such as night terrors or sleepwalking, are classified as a sleep disturbance, but if your child is not wakened from the event, he will fall back asleep and not remember the episode in the morning. Although your child's nighttime sleep appears to be disrupted, he may not be affected during the day. However, your sleep may be disturbed because you will be wakened by your child's arousal.

Sleep Disorder Classifications

There are three types of common sleep disorders in children. The disorders discussed in this book are either type 1 or type 2.

1. Disorders that cause insomnias or excessive sleepiness. Doctors call these problems dyssomnias. Insomnia includes disorders that cause difficulty falling asleep, staying asleep, or waking too early in the morning, as well as problems with the timing of sleep. In addition to experiencing difficulty falling and staying asleep at night, there will be other effects of this sleep disturbance, which may include your child experiencing excessive sleepiness during the day or feeling some effect of the insomnia in his daytime functioning — for example, in school performance, behavior, mood, memory, or learning.

2. Disorders that lead to unusual behaviors or experiences or feelings (such as sleepwalking or nightmares) while sleeping. Doctors call these problems parasomnias.

3. Disorders of sleep that are part of other medical or psychiatric problems. There are many health problems that can include sleep disturbances. For example, if your child has bad eczema, she may not be able to sleep because of her dry, itchy skin.

Did You Know?

Type 3 Sleep Problem
If you think your child has a type 3 sleep problem associated with a medical or psychiatric problem, you should consult with your doctor.

SLEEP DISORDER CHARACTERISTICS

The signs and symptoms of sleep disorders are not always easy to detect or delineate because there are many different varieties of sleep disturbance. However, the characteristics of sleep disorders tend to fall into 'either/or' categories.

Sleep disturbances can be:
- *Either* easily recognized *or* difficult to recognize. An easily recognized problem is a child who resists bedtime, falls asleep too late, and gets inadequate sleep. A problem that may not be recognized is the child who snores loudly and persistently and displays daytime fatigue from sleep apnea.

- *Either* temporary (only lasting nights to weeks, such as sleep disruption at the time of stress) *or* chronic (lasting months to years).

- *Either* problematic for the child only *or* problematic for parents or the whole family.

- *Either* acquired (which means the child was not born with the problem but developed it with time) *or* inherited (which means passed through the genes from parent to child).

- *Either* related to both NREM and REM sleep states (bruxism or teeth grinding occurs in both sleep states, for example) *or* occur in particular states (nightmares occur in REM dreaming sleep, for example).

- *Either* easily treated (by using behavioral techniques, for example) *or* difficult to treat (requiring surgery or medication, for example).

- *Either* have one preferred solution (removing your child's tonsils and adenoids to treat sleep apnea, for example) *or* several solutions (teaching your child to sleep through the night, for example).

Family Context

Textbook definitions of sleep disorders are complicated by the family context. Depending on the family's expectations, a child with the same sleep habits may be seen in one family as a problem sleeper and in another as a normal sleeper. For example, if you and your partner tend to be 'night owls' and prefer a late bedtime and rise time, you can imagine the problem if your child is a 'morning lark' who prefers the opposite schedule. Your child's sleep patterns would not fit with your schedule and needs.

However, the same child with the identical sleep patterns would not be considered a problem sleeper if he lived in another family where both his parents also preferred a 'lark' schedule with early bedtimes and rise times. What is a sleep disorder for one family may not be seen as a problem for another family.

Examples of Childhood Sleep Disorder by Types

Type 1	Type 2	Type 3
Dyssomnias that cause insomnia, difficulty falling asleep, staying asleep, waking too early in the morning, or causing excessive daytime sleepiness:	Parasomnias that lead to unusual behaviors or experiences or feelings while sleeping:	Disorders that are part of other medical or psychiatric problems:
Inadequate sleep hygiene	Confusional arousals Night terrors Sleepwalking	Associated with psychiatric disorders, such as mood or anxiety disorders — e.g. difficulty falling asleep in children with anxiety disorder
Limit-setting sleep disorder	Sleep talking	Associated with neurologic disorders, such as sleep-related epilepsy (seizures)
Sleep-onset association disorder	Rhythmic movement disorder	Associated with other medical disorders, such as sleep-related asthma
Nocturnal eating (drinking) syndrome	Nightmares	
Circadian rhythm sleep disorders (delayed or advanced sleep phase syndrome)	Bruxism (teeth grinding)	
Obstructive sleep apnea syndrome	Enuresis (bed-wetting)	
Narcolepsy		
Restless legs syndrome		

Did You Know?

Shared Concerns

Sleep studies show that in many different countries, one out of four children are identified by their parents as having a sleep problem. Across cultures, the most commonly reported problems relating to behavioral sleep disturbances are difficulty getting children to bed at night and problems with children who wake up frequently throughout the night.

Cultural Context

We have little knowledge about different cultural issues and their impact on children's sleep, except in the areas of co-sleeping and bedtime rituals. We do know that some cultures have well-established expectations for bedtime routines and others have unstructured and flexible bedtimes. We also know that there are more children in the world who co-sleep in the same bed as their parents or in the same room than who sleep in a separate bedroom. Even industrialized societies, such as Japan, and not just less industrialized societies, promote co-sleeping. Because of the increasing migration of families throughout the world and the inter-marriage between cultural groups, parents are often faced with a question of which sleep culture to follow — old country or new country, mother's culture or father's culture.

If you and your partner have different cultural backgrounds, you will need to discuss your expectations for sleep behavior in your child and choose a consistent practice of parenting around sleep issues.

---

case history: **Sammy**

Sammy and his parents, Anna and Tom, came to our office to discuss Sammy's problem with sleeping. Their concern was that Sammy resisted going to sleep at the bedtime they chose, at 8:00 p.m., with the apparent result that he had trouble getting up early enough in the morning to get to day care on time. He would fight, cry, and generally become difficult when it came to bedtime and would not fall asleep in his room by himself.

Each evening, Anna and Tom would give in after 1 to 2 hours of struggling, and let Sammy join them in the living room. When Sammy was allowed to stay up with his parents watching television, he would eventually fall asleep around 10:00 p.m. without any fuss. Despite trying various strategies they had read about in magazine articles, Anna and Tom were not successful in changing this pattern. They felt that Sammy was not getting enough sleep because of this bedtime resistance and, consequently, was tired during the day.

We explained that according to the International Classification of Sleep Disorders (which is how sleep experts define different types of sleep disturbance), Sammy would fit into the first category of disorders, with a disorder that causes difficulty falling asleep. His disorder would be called a limit-setting sleep disorder because Anna and Tom are unable to take charge in the evening and consistently get Sammy into bed and asleep at the time that they expect. Sammy is displaying problems from his sleep disorder because he is fatigued during the day.

We also explained that Sammy's problem was, in part, relative. If Sammy had parents who believed that it is more important to have children participate in socializing at night, for example, who prefer that their children not fall asleep in their own room, and who do not take their children to day care in the morning, then they might let him fall asleep in the living room at 10:00 p.m. and sleep later in the morning. If Sammy were raised in this family, he would not be viewed as having a sleep disorder. Sammy might present problems with limits during the day, but he would still not have a sleep disorder. In fact, in this family, Sammy might be able to fall asleep at an earlier bedtime without 2 hours of fussing, either in the living room or in bed with a sibling or parent.

This does not imply that it is wrong for Anna and Tom to want Sammy to learn to fall asleep alone at a regular time according to their schedule. To achieve this desired behavior, Anna and Tom have to learn how to set a bedtime routine and teach Sammy to fall asleep alone. This will allow Sammy to get adequate sleep and to be well-rested during the day.

SLEEP DISORDER CONSEQUENCES

- If children or adults do not get enough sleep, some of the consequences can include difficulty with memory, learning, emotions, behavior, and relationships with friends.

- When children are sleep deprived, they may not look tired during the day, but may be irritable and inattentive.

- Children who do not sleep well are more likely to become adults who do not sleep well.

- Mothers of children who do not sleep well are more likely to be depressed.

Sleep Disorders through the Ages

Infants (Age 6 to 12 months)

Settling at night and frequent waking are the most common problems of sleep in infants. These same problems can continue into toddler and childhood ages.

Q. When should I take my infant to the doctor with a sleep problem?

A. See your doctor if your child shows the following signs and symptoms:

- If, in addition to problems sleeping, you notice any other health problems, such as frequent or forceful vomiting, breathing difficulties, blue spells, or difficulty feeding

- If the sleep pattern is not improving (including more sleep at night and longer sleep periods) after the age of 3 months

- If your baby does not seem to have periods when he is well rested, playful, and alert

- If your child continues to have his days and nights mixed up after the first few months of life

- If you are unable to cope with your own sleep deprivation, depression, or exhaustion

- If your child has a medical problem (for example, eczema) that is interfering with his sleep

Common Sleep Problems in Infants (Age 6 to 12 months)

Problem	Characteristics
Nocturnal eating (drinking) syndrome	Your baby may be so accustomed to eating through the night (either from breast-feeding or bottle-feeding) that he cannot sleep through the night because of this pattern. This common problem is called a nocturnal eating (drinking) syndrome. Remember that this is a relative problem — an acceptable pattern for a child in some families and one that parents want to change in others.
Sleep-onset association disorder	Your baby has not yet learned to fall back asleep on his own when he wakes up naturally at night. Some babies learn this naturally, and some need your help. Sleep experts call this a sleep-onset association disorder.
Delayed or advanced sleep phase syndrome	Your baby may have trouble sleeping if his sleep/wake schedule is chronically delayed (for example, if he has late afternoon naps, he will have trouble falling asleep at bedtime) or advanced.
Rhythmic movement disorder	Your child may develop rhythmic movements (such as head-banging or body-rocking) as he transitions from wake to sleep. This movement may disturb you, but does not disturb your child's sleep.
Pain at night (teething, ear infection, heartburn)	Sleep may be delayed or disrupted in your baby when he starts teething at 5 to 8 months, although this should be only for the few days when his teeth are erupting. Other causes of pain at night, such as an ear infection or heartburn in babies with acid reflux, can disrupt sleep.
Separation anxiety	Your baby may have difficulty settling at night due to the development of separation anxiety, which is usually seen after the age of 9 months.
Poor hygiene (sleep environment)	Your baby may have difficulty sleeping if the bedroom environment is too noisy, light, cold, or warm.

Toddlers and Preschoolers (Age 1 to 5 Years)

The most common behavioral sleep disturbances in the toddler and preschool years are behavioral in origin. Bedtime struggles and frequent night waking are a common complaint of parents with children in this age group. These problems lead to insufficient nighttime sleep and daytime fatigue in your child.

Common Sleep Problems in Toddlers and Preschoolers (Age 1 to 5)

Problem	Characteristics
Poor schedule and hygiene	By this age, your child may have developed difficulties settling at night due to an irregular schedule and poor sleep hygiene.
Settling and waking disorders	Your toddler or preschooler may have the same difficulties as infants in settling at night and waking frequently, which can lead to insufficient sleep. These problems may be also due to nocturnal eating (drinking) syndrome, sleep onset association disorder, or a sleep phase disturbance (sleeping and waking at a delayed or advanced time), as described in the younger child.
Rhythmic movement disorder	Your toddler or preschooler may continue to have rhythmic movements although these usually resolve by 4 years of age.
Nighttime fears, anxiety, and nightmares	Your child may delay sleep due to bedtime fears and anxiety. At this age, he may experience more nightmares.
Limit-setting disorder	Now that your child can get out of bed, difficulty settling at night may be related to limit-setting problems if your child makes bedtime demands, such as asking for one more story or one more drink before settling in. If these requests are not satisfied, he may refuse to stay in bed.

Q. **When should I take my toddler or preschooler to the doctor with a sleep problem?**

A. See your doctor for evaluation if your toddler or preschooler shows the following signs and symptoms:

- If you are concerned about any of the medical problems or pain that may be interfering with your child's sleep

- If your child has persistent and loud snoring or experiences pauses or any difficulty with breathing during sleep

- If your child appears to be getting enough sleep at night, but seems cranky, irritable, hyperactive, inattentive, or sleepy during the day

- If your child displays excessive anxiety about separating from you both during the day and at night

- If your child was previously a good sleeper but now has recently developed a problem with sleep

- If your child is not able to transition from two naps to one nap a day

- If night terrors, sleepwalking, or nightmares are occurring frequently

Common Sleep Problems in Toddlers and Preschoolers (Age 1 to 5) *(continued...)*	
Problem	**Characteristics**
Night terrors and sleepwalking	Your child may develop night terrors and sleepwalking episodes that may appear to disturb his sleep, but may not cause him any daytime symptoms of fatigue.
Sleep apnea	Your child may develop at this age other sleep disturbances, such as central or obstructive sleep apnea, that do cause daytime symptoms of fatigue.

School-Age Children (Age 5 to 12)

Children between the ages of 5 and 12 can be good sleepers. They should go to sleep easily, sleep continuously through the night, and wake up spontaneously in the morning without much difficulty. During the day, at this age, children should be alert and energetic without the need for a daytime nap. Despite this natural ability for good sleep, many children continue to have sleep problems at this age.

There are two types of sleep problems seen in the school years. One type includes the children who had sleep disturbance at an earlier age, whether it was behavioral in origin, such as a limit-setting disorder, or acquired but not yet recognized, such as obstructive sleep apnea syndrome. The other type is children who develop new sleep disturbances that were not present or present but not problematic before the school-age years, such as enuresis.

Q. When should I take my school-age child to the doctor with a sleep problem?

A. See your doctor for evaluation if your child was previously a good sleeper without any evidence of daytime fatigue and develops the following symptoms:

- If your child's teacher complains of daytime fatigue in your child despite your impression that he is getting adequate sleep

- If there is a new onset of an arousal disorder (night terrors, sleepwalking) that your child did not develop before the age of 6 to 7 years

- If your child develops the need for a regular daytime nap

- If your child demonstrates evidence of a sleep disorder with loud snoring, pauses in his breathing, or extreme restlessness at night

Common Sleep Problems in School-Age Children (Age 5 to 12)

Problem	Characteristics
Sleep problems present at earlier ages	
Poor schedule and hygiene	Your child may have ongoing difficulties settling at night if he has never developed a regular sleep/wake schedule and continues to have poor sleep hygiene.
Settling and waking problems	Your school-age child may have the same difficulties as younger children in settling at night and waking frequently, which can lead to insufficient sleep. These problems may also be due to sleep-onset association disorder or a sleep phase disturbance (sleeping and waking at a delayed or advanced time). It is much less common at this age to have ongoing problems with eating or drinking at night.
Nighttime fears, anxieties, and nightmares	Your child may continue to delay sleep due to nightime fears and anxiety. Nightmares may continue to be a problem.
Limit-setting disorder	Your child may continue to have a limit-setting disorder, making frequent demands at night and refusing to stay in bed.
Night terrors and sleepwalking	By school age, if he had an arousal disorder of night terrors or sleepwalking, this should have resolved. In some children, it can continue into the school-age years, but should be less frequent. This problem is of more concern if it starts at this age.
Obstructive sleep apnea syndrome	Earlier symptoms of obstructive sleep apnea may not have been recognized or may appear in school-age children for the first time.
Sleep problems present for the first time in the school-age years	
Bed-wetting (enuresis)	Your child may have bed-wetting episodes which would have been a part of normal development at younger ages.
Restless legs syndrome	Your child will have unusual sensations in his legs at night, which delay sleep onset, and he may have involuntary leg kicking during sleep.

Adolescents (Age 12 to 18)

The most common sleep disorders among adolescents are an irregular schedule and lack of adequate sleep at night. The most common reason for fatigue in adolescents is insufficient sleep. The amount of sleep needed changes as children grow, but adolescents still need more sleep than adults. These sleep problems in adolescence can be resolved with changes to sleep hygiene by establishing a sleep schedule and increasing the time for sleep. However, this is a challenge at this age because of the demands on teenagers to accommodate school, work, and social activities, and difficulties parents have in setting limits and controls.

Causes of Adolescent Sleep Problems (Age 12 to 18 years)

Problem	Characteristics
Insufficient sleep	Your teenager experiences problems caused by insufficient sleep, most commonly inadequate time in bed. Another common problem resulting in insufficient sleep at this age is the development of a preference for a delayed sleep schedule, falling asleep and waking at a later than desired schedule. Other causes for insufficient sleep include an irregular sleep/wake schedule and poor sleep hygiene. Finally, your teenager may be having difficulty sleeping due to depression or anxiety, or he may have developed an adult-type insomnia called primary insomnia, which is a diagnosis made when all the above problems are not the cause of the insomnia.
Fragmented sleep	Your teenager may have fragmented sleep and many arousals from sleep at night caused by sleep disorders, medical or psychiatric disorders, or the effect of substances, such as nicotine, alcohol, and drugs, or the effect of drug withdrawal. Restless legs syndrome can cause sleep-onset insomnia and disturbed sleep, but is considered rare in children and adolescents.
Increased need for sleep	Your adolescent has an increased need for sleep associated with temporary illness, depression, or the use of illicit drugs.
Narcolepsy	Narcolepsy, a rare sleep disorder, can start in adolescence, with excessive daytime sleepiness, and not be recognized until later in adult life.

Q. When should I take my teenager to the doctor with a sleep problem?

A. In the teenage years, it is important to identify who is concerned about sleep or daytime alertness. There may be times when you are very worried about your teenager, but she does not seem to recognize the problem. At other times, your teenager will initiate the need to seek help. See your doctor if your teenager shows the following signs and symptoms:

- If your teenager is excessively sleepy during the day
- If your teenager's school performance decreases
- If you suspect your teenager may have mood disturbance (which can be both caused by or causing the sleep problems)
- If your teenager has a motor vehicle accident or other problems caused by daytime sleepiness
- If you or your teenager have any other concerns about his sleep or daytime performance

Chapter 2

Treatment of Sleep Disorders

T HERE ARE MANY DIFFERENT types of sleep disturbances, problems, syndromes, and disorders. Not surprisingly, there are many different treatment strategies depending on the child's specific disturbance.

Education

Learning as much as you can about healthy sleep habits and sleep disorders from reading books and discussing issues with your health-care provider is the best first treatment. Involve your child in this education process, especially your older child or teenager, so she can take control of her own sleep health. Let other caregivers and teachers know about any sleep problems your child may be experiencing, and give them the information they need to support treatment. This will create a consistent approach in dealing with the sleep issues.

Educating yourself about sleep should include learning about the basics of sleep biology, the prevention of sleep problems, the promotion of good sleep hygiene, and the problems and solutions to sleep problems. With this education, you will be successful at resolving many childhood sleep problems.

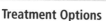

Did You Know?

Treatment Options
The treatment of sleep problems depends on the specific disorder. In children, the treatment is often based on two basic approaches — parent education and behavioral intervention. For some sleep disorders, other treatment options are used, including surgery, dental or breathing appliances for airway obstruction, or, less commonly, medication.

Behavioral Intervention

In this treatment option, parents learn new ways to manage their children's behavior around sleep. Behavioral intervention is the most frequent treatment used for children because most sleep disturbances in children are the result of a behavioral cause.

Because there is not one type of behavioral treatment that is the most effective in all cases, knowing the various options is important. Regardless of which option you choose, you need to carry it out on a consistent basis. If it doesn't work, it is most likely that you have not been consistent, rather than it being the 'wrong' treatment.

Behavioral Treatment Options

Two primary behavioral modification options are extinction and positive routines/faded bedtime. Here's how these treatments would apply to the problems of settling down at bedtime and frequent waking in an infant. These treatment strategies will be described in more detail in the following chapters as they relate to particular sleep problems.

Extinction

Extinction is also called the 'cold turkey' method. Using this method, you would, for example, simply decide that you are not going to respond to your child's frequent requests at bedtime and during the night, buy some good earplugs, and let your child 'cry it out' until he learns to sleep through the night on his own. There are other variations to the method of extinction, which are more acceptable to families and more effective in dealing with sleep issues.

Graduated Extinction

To achieve the goal of settling in and sleeping through the night, a more gradual approach can be used. Gradual extinction is the approach recommended in this book and by many sleep experts for progressively teaching your child how to sleep through the night in a supportive, yet firm manner. You do this by ignoring your child's inappropriate behavior for increasing lengths of time, while continuing to check on him.

Extinction with Parental Presence

While few of the behavioral intervention methods for dealing with sleep problems have been studied extensively in a scientific way, extinction with parental presence has been studied even less than the others. In this method, the parent sleeps in the child's room and ignores the child's inappropriate behavior. The parent does this for 1 week and then resumes sleeping away from the child. This may be a useful method for an anxious child to decrease temporarily his tension around bedtime and his sleep disturbance.

Positive Routines/Faded Bedtime

Similar to the behavioral treatment of adults with insomnia, this strategy is used when children have difficulty settling at bedtime. It involves teaching good bedtime routines and delaying bedtime so that your child learns to fall asleep quickly. Once your child has learned to fall asleep quickly at a later bedtime, you gradually move the bedtime earlier until you arrive at the desired time.

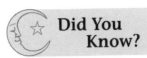

Did You Know?

Cold Turkey
Although the cold turkey method will work in some cases, many families do not prefer the extinction treatment because it may cause their child to become very distressed, making it difficult to carry through in a consistent manner. The parent will naturally feel compelled to give in. This method is especially not suggested for the infant or toddler who is breast-feeding or bottle-feeding through the night.

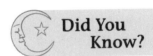

Did You Know?

Positive, Not Punitive
The methods recommended in this book for resolving behavioral-based sleep problems use positive reinforcement of consequences but are not punitive. You may be concerned about upsetting your child by enforcing rules about sleep, setting limits at bedtime, and gently teaching your child that he can fall asleep alone at night. However, it is known that children need and indeed like to have these types of limits and parental controls. Rather than causing problems, it increases their feelings of security.

SLEEP DIARY

Part of educating yourself about sleep includes understanding your own child's sleep patterns. A sleep diary can be helpful for this purpose.

There are several reasons to document your child's current sleep/wake cycle over several weeks:

- Sometimes simply putting this into writing and then reviewing the diary will allow you to see what the problem is and how to start to correct it – for example, if your child has a very irregular sleep/wake schedule.

- A sleep diary can help your health-care provider understand what is happening at home when you meet with her to discuss your child's sleep problems.

- A sleep diary is helpful for gauging the progress of a behavioral sleep program. This is similar to the feedback you would get from keeping track of your weight if you were on a diet program. You would be motivated to continue the program when you could compare your baseline weight to the weight loss after sticking to a diet regime. In the same way, you may be motivated to continue your sleep program with your child when you can see in the diaries that things are improving. Alternatively, if your child's sleep is not improving, you can show the before and after diaries to your health-care provider for further assistance.

Instructions

A sleep diary is very simple to compile. Follow these instructions as you complete the diary on the next page.

1. Complete it for at least two continuous weeks to see your child's sleep pattern over time.

2. Each day, write down the time your child went to bed, how often he woke up and for how long, the time he woke in the morning, and when he slept during the day, if applicable.

3. Don't bother to fill it in during the night when you are tired. Each morning, you can complete the diary based on how many times your child woke and for how long.

4. Note when your child is in bed, using an arrow pointing downwards (↓)

5. Note when your child is out of bed, using an arrow pointing upwards (↑)

6. Fill in the squares when your child is sleeping.

7. Use the comments section to write down information about your child's sleep during the night – for example, nightmares, sleepwalking episodes, any difficulty settling, snacks or drinks at bedtime or during the night. Also note positive changes that you want to remember.

8. Make extra copies of this form for compiling sleep diaries in subsequent weeks.

Sleep Diary

Name:_____   Date:_____

Date	Day	6 p.m.	7	8	9	10	11	12	1 a.m.	2	3	4	5	6	7	8	9	10	11	12	1 p.m.	2	3	4	5
e.g.					↓						↑	↓				↑									
	1																								
	2																								
	3																								
	4																								
	5																								
	6																								
	7																								
	8																								
	9																								
	10																								
	11																								
	12																								
	13																								
	14																								

Date	Day	Comment
e.g.		Nightmare at 3:30 a.m.
	1	
	2	
	3	
	4	
	5	
	6	
	7	
	8	
	9	
	10	
	11	
	12	
	13	
	14	

Medications

It may be tempting at night, when you have had too many sleepless nights because of your sleepless child, to pull out some medicine with sleepiness as a side effect and solve your child's problem with drugs. If these are your thoughts, you are not alone. We know from parent surveys that it is not uncommon for parents to use over-the-counter medication to improve their child's sleep with and without the knowledge of their child's doctor. In addition, parents also receive prescriptions from their child's doctor to improve sleep.

However, neither of these practices is supported by scientific research. Although medications can be used to allow you and your child to get a few nights of sleep, the medication's effect will not last and has potential harmful side effects.

In healthy, typically developing children, it is unlikely that medication should be used at all. These sleep problems can be addressed by better understanding the reason for the disturbance, improving sleep hygiene, and using the behavioral techniques described in this book and other sleep literature.

case history: John

Patsy and Brian came to our clinic with concerns about their son's sleep. John is 5 years old, the youngest of four siblings. Patsy and Brian did not have trouble getting their older three children to sleep, but it seems like a never-ending battle with John at bedtime. He wants to stay up as late as his 10-, 12-, and 14-year-old brothers.

In an effort to understand this problem, Patsy and Brian read many sleep articles in parenting magazines and surfed the Net for relevant information, but still have had no luck settling John at bedtime. They became so upset that they have decided to try some over-the-counter medication recommended to them by a colleague at work. When John was given just a small dose of Gravol (dimenhydrinate) he fell asleep quickly and there were no bedtime battles. But after 2 weeks, this medication no longer seemed to be have the same effect. They came to our clinic to discuss if it is safe to increase the dose and how long can they give it to John without causing any problems.

We counseled them that this type of sleep treatment is not recommended. As soon as John stops taking the medicine, he will revert back to the same pattern of having difficulty settling at night. He can also develop a tolerance to this type of medicine, and eventually he will need larger doses (which can have side effects, such as causing morning drowsiness) to have the same effect. The real problem – his parents' failure to set limits for John and have him fall asleep while his older siblings are still awake – has not been addressed.

PARENTAL ADVICE ON MEDICATIONS FOR SLEEP PROBLEMS FROM THE AMERICAN ACADEMY OF SLEEP MEDICINE

A recent task force published in the medical literature in 2005 and supported by the American Academy of Sleep Medicine made the following recommendations about the use of drugs in the treatment of childhood insomnia:

1. Your doctor must evaluate your child's sleep problem carefully to determine the exact cause before suggesting medication.

2. If you have an infant or young child who is healthy and developing normally, it is very rare to need sleep medication.

3. Your doctor should discuss other strategies for improving your child's sleep. Even if you and your doctor are considering sleep medications, they will not work to solve the problem if not used in combination with other strategies, such as behavioral intervention, educating yourself about normal sleep patterns, and sleep hygiene.

4. You must make sure to correct all the possible sleep hygiene problems with your child before considering medication.

5. You must have a clear goal as to your expectations from the medication and discuss with your doctor how long your child will be on medication.

6. You should only use sleep medication for a short term.

7. If you are considering giving medication to your teenager, ensure that he is not also using any alcohol or drugs, and if it is your daughter, do not give any medications if there is a chance that she is pregnant. Some of the medications would have harmful side effects to fetal development.

8. You must tell your doctor about any herbal products or over-the-counter products that you are giving to your child for sleep or other problems.

9. You need to know about the possible side effects of the medication so you know what to watch for.

Drug Treatment Conditions

Even though there is not enough scientific research on medicating children with sleep difficulties, it does not imply that there is no role for medication in all children. There are specific conditions that respond well to drug treatments, often prescribed in conjunction with behavioral treatments.

Common Prescription Sleep Medications for Children
- Chloral hydrate
- Clonidine
- Benzodiazepine
- Antidepressants

Did You Know?

Sleep Prescriptions
Many doctors recommend the use of prescription and over-the-counter sleep aid products frequently. A survey in the United States revealed that more than 75% of pediatricians had recommended a nonprescription medication for sleep and more than 50% had prescribed a sleep medication at least once in the 6 months before the survey.

Restless Legs Syndrome

For example, the treatment of restless legs syndrome, a sleep disturbance caused by involuntary leg movements at night leading to daytime fatigue, may involve medications, in addition to optimizing sleep hygiene and obtaining adequate sleep. Drugs can act on the neurotransmitters (chemicals in the brain) responsible for this sleep disorder.

Delayed Sleep Phase Syndrome

Another condition where medication may be used is for adolescents with delayed sleep phase syndrome. Your doctor may prescribe medication or suggest melatonin in addition to other interventions.

Acute Stress

Short-term use of sleep medications may also be prescribed when there is an acute stress — for example, if your child is not sleeping because he is hospitalized, has a medical problem, or feels acutely stressed due to a family crisis.

Special Needs

Sleep medications may be prescribed for a short term in combination with behavioral interventions to children with special needs, such as developmental delay, attention deficit/hyperactivity disorder, autism, or other medical, psychiatric, or developmental disabilities.

Side Effects

If you are considering using medications to help your child sleep, you should be aware of several potential problems. Some medications have significant potential side effects, such as causing excessive daytime sleepiness. In addition, your child may get used to the sedating effects of the drug, and it will become ineffective. When the drug is withdrawn from your child, his sleep problems may recur or may even worsen.

Melatonin

We naturally produce the hormone melatonin in darkness. It is excreted by the pineal gland in the brain. Melatonin has an important role in the regulation of our circadian rhythm (our internal biological clock) that keeps us adjusted to a 24-hour day-night cycle.

RECOMMENDATIONS FOR MEDICATION TREATMENTS

- Before giving any over-the-counter sleep medication to your child, discuss this with your doctor.

- Before using medications to treat your child's sleep problem, remember that there are no definitive studies to guide your doctor about drug effectiveness, safety, or even choice if your child is healthy and developing normally, but has problems going to sleep and sleeping through the night.

- Before using over-the-counter or prescription medications, try improving sleep hygiene and make behavioral changes to improve your child's sleep.

- For some children with specific sleep disorders (such as restless legs syndrome) who do not respond to non-pharmacological treatment, medications may be indicated. For children with special needs, who do not respond to behavioral changes alone, the addition of sleep medications for short periods of time may be useful. You should talk to your doctor if you have these concerns about your child.

For Use in Adults

Melatonin promotes the onset of sleep and can be used to induce sleep when given in much larger doses than our bodies would naturally produce. Melatonin is known to be useful in the treatment of adults with sleep disturbance, such as delayed sleep phase syndrome, jet lag syndrome, and desynchronized sleep (not adjusted to a schedule) due to shift work.

For Use in Children

When children are given melatonin, it will have the effect (in most cases) of making them sleepy. However, the effect of melatonin will only last a short time. That is, melatonin will help children to fall asleep, but not to stay asleep through the night.

In the treatment of children who are having trouble initiating sleep because of a problem with the timing of sleep (delayed sleep phase syndrome), melatonin may be effective, but in children it has not been rigorously studied for this use. We do not know what the possible effects on children in the future may be who are given an extra large dose of a natural hormone that is only produced in humans in small quantities. Despite the limitations in the research studies, doctors do use melatonin for children, especially for children with special needs to help them fall asleep and for blind children.

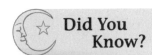

Did You Know?

Melatonin Dose
If you give your child melatonin, you are giving him a 'natural' product in an 'unnatural' dosage. Your child will receive a much larger amount than he would naturally produce. While the long-term safety is not scientifically known, the large amount of hormone may cause problems with the onset of puberty, for example, or other problems that we don't currently know.

Although melatonin is available over the counter in the United States and Canada, due to the lack of research in healthy children with sleep problems and the possible side effects, you should discuss its use with your doctor and learn about the latest research before giving it to your child.

Other Treatment Options

Bright-Light Therapy

Bright-light therapy involves exposing your child to artificial intense light in the morning to help reset the body's rhythms. A more natural way of doing this, which is often recommended by sleep doctors for problems with the timing of sleep, is to ensure exposure to natural sunlight in the morning. This recommendation may be given for children with a delayed sleep phase. Although bright-light therapy has been studied in adults, currently there is no evidence of the safety and efficacy of this treatment in children.

Alarm Systems for Bed-wetting

Children who wet the bed may sleep with an alarm that wakens them with the first episode of dampness to decrease bed-wetting.

Surgery

Surgery to the airways, especially to remove the tonsils and adenoids, which can block the airway and lead to obstruction during sleep, is the most common treatment for obstructive sleep apnea syndrome in childhood.

Breathing or Dental Appliances

Children who have difficulty breathing during sleep, called obstructive sleep apnea, sometimes need to sleep with a machine that produces a constant flow and pressure of air to the airway to keep air passages open during sleep. This is very common for adults, but can also be used as a treatment for children with sleep-related breathing problems.

A dental appliance, which is worn over the teeth to keep the upper airway open during sleep, is commonly used in adults, but not commonly in children, with obstructive sleep apnea syndrome.

PART 3

Step-by-Step Guide to Better Sleep

CHAPTER 1 Childhood Insomnia (Sleeplessness)......... 88

CHAPTER 2 Nocturnal Eating (Drinking) Syndrome 94

CHAPTER 3 Sleep-Onset Association Disorder.......... 106

CHAPTER 4 Limit-Setting Disorder 125

CHAPTER 5 Circadian Rhythm Sleep Disorders
(Delayed and Advanced Sleep Phase Syndrome) .. 132

CHAPTER 6 Excessive Crying.......................... 149

CHAPTER 7 Confusional Arousals, Night Terrors,
and Sleepwalking................................. 158

CHAPTER 8 Nightmares and Nighttime Anxiety 168

CHAPTER 9 Snoring, Apnea, and Hypoventilation........ 178

CHAPTER 10 Bed-Wetting (Enuresis).................... 192

CHAPTER 11 Restless Legs Syndrome 199

CHAPTER 12 Teeth Grinding and Gnashing (Bruxism) ... 208

CHAPTER 13 Rhythmic Movement Disorder............. 213

CHAPTER 14 Narcolepsy 218

CHAPTER 15 Teenage Sleepiness...................... 226

CHAPTER 16 Sleep during Pregnancy 235

Chapter 1

Childhood Insomnia (Sleeplessness)

INSOMNIA (SLEEPLESSNESS) IS the most common sleep problem of childhood, from infancy to early adolescence, characterized by difficulty settling at night, sleeping through the night, and waking too early in the morning. Insomnia is not one disorder but a symptom that can be caused by many different problems. In children, insomnia is most commonly caused by behavioral problems and leads to insufficient sleep and a tired child. As a result, your child may experience problems during the day with memory, attention, or learning.

What Causes Childhood Insomnia?

There are four main behavioral causes of childhood insomnia. It is not uncommon for a child to have a combination of more than one of these problems; in fact, he may even have a combination of all four of these common causes. In that case, the approach to improving sleep is to deal with one issue at a time — and to know where to start.

Nocturnal Eating (Drinking) Disorder

Don't be alarmed to read that your beautiful baby who loves to breast-feed or bottle-feed all night long may have a nocturnal eating (drinking) disorder. This ominous name is given to one of the common causes of sleeplessness in young babies and toddlers who wake frequently at night to quench their thirst. Later in life, some adults have a similar disorder where they wake to eat, which is why the name of the disorder includes both eating and drinking.

After the age of 6 months, a healthy baby can learn to consume enough calories and his tummy is large enough to hold enough fluids that he doesn't need to wake frequently for a refill. However, many young babies just get used to drinking more often, and then it becomes a habit that you can help him change. Some families are happy to continue this pattern until their baby eventually starts to stretch out the nighttime feeds. Other families want to help their babies to adjust their eating times so that they drink more during the daytime and learn to sleep through the night.

Sleep-Onset Association Disorder

How your child does or doesn't fall asleep can be a problem, especially if falling asleep requires an 'association' with your help in some way. Some of the things we associate with falling asleep are helpful, and some are not. Associations with falling asleep that can be problematic include the presence of a parent, a specific bed that is not your child's own, music, or a pacifier. If these associations are present when your child falls asleep at bedtime, but not at periods of natural waking during the night, your child may have difficulty falling back asleep on his own. You may find yourself having to wake up at night to recreate the same associations as when he fell asleep the first time to help him return to sleep.

Limit-Setting Sleep Disorder

Do you find that your child wants to be in charge? This may happen both during the day and in the evening, particularly at bedtime. Many children like to test the limits and see what control they can have over their parents. This is a natural part of growing up. When your child checks out what limits you set, he is also learning about respect, authority, and control. As he develops, you gradually give him more control, which he earns with his developing maturity.

However, sometimes you cannot get your child to sleep because you have not learned to set limits about sleep properly. This results in him getting inadequate sleep. It may be harder to set limits in the evening when you are tired, or perhaps you and your partner do not always agree on what the limits should be or how they should be enforced. When it seems like your child is in charge and you are unable to elicit his cooperation to get him to sleep at night, he has a limit-setting sleep disorder. You will recognize this easily when you try to leave him in his bed to fall asleep alone. There are frequent demands for more stories, more songs, more water, more trips to the bathroom…you name it.

Sleep-Timing Disorders

There are times when we feel more or less sleepy during the day and night. When your child develops a pattern where her sleep-wake pattern is too early or too late, then she has adjusted her biologic clock. When the sleep preference is later, your child goes to bed later than you want and wakes up later — a common teenage sleep problem. The sleep preference can also be earlier, usually in a younger child who falls asleep soon after dinner and wakens early in the morning, even before the sun rises. These sleep patterns cause insomnia. If one of these patterns is well established, you need to recognize it and slowly help your child adapt to a normal schedule.

Childhood Vs. Adult Insomnia Factors

There are many differences between insomnia or sleeplessness in adults and children, the chief one being that adults recognize when they have insomnia and may feel anxious about this problem, thus compounding their sleeplessness. When children cannot get to sleep, stay asleep, or wake early in the morning, their parents may be anxious about this pattern, but they may not realize that their behavior is problematic.

Factors	Adult	Child
Cause	Variety of causes, including stress and depression	Most often behavioral cause
Responsibility	The adult cannot sleep and is usually anxious about it The adult wants to go to sleep at night	The parents recognize the problem but the child suffers the consequences of inadequate sleep and cranky parents The child wants to stay up at night
Insight into problem	The adult understands need for sleep	The young child has no insight into the problem
Motivation to change	High	Low to none
Control over the problem regarding schedules, hygiene, regularity, etc.	Adult is able to choose time for bedtime/wake, sleep environment, regularity, and other sleep hygiene issues	Child does not have control over this issue Parents choose time for bedtime/wake, sleep environment, regularity, and other sleep hygiene issues
Treatment strategies	Behavioral with or without medication	Usually only behavioral treatment
Outcome	Can be good, but often a chronic problem	Excellent chance for resolution of the problem

case study: **Heather**

Martha and Gary are tired first-time parents of a healthy baby girl. Their daughter, Heather, is 11 months old and is a joy in every way – during the day, that is. However, both parents are exhausted because of her poor sleep patterns at night.

The first few months after she was born were difficult ones because Martha had to return to work when Heather was 3 months old. It's been hard to adjust to parenting and working. Martha is committed to nursing Heather, and she feeds her before leaving for work in the morning, expresses milk and stores it for the following day while at work, nurses her as soon as she gets home, and then through the night. Heather seems to nurse more from 7:00 p.m. when Martha gets home until 7:00 a.m when she leaves, drinking less from the bottle during the day. She seems to be getting the majority of her calories at night instead of during the day. Sometimes, Heather will waken every 2 to 3 hours at night, which means she can be awake up to five times during the night.

Heather also cannot fall asleep without being nursed or rocked. If Martha tries to put Heather back into her crib when she is not fully asleep, she will waken and cry vigorously until either Martha nurses her again or Gary gets out of bed and rocks Heather gently to sleep. Martha and Gary are exhausted but they recognize that things could be worse. Their next door neighbor with a similar age baby has to take the baby for rides around town at night to get him to fall asleep because he will only fall asleep in the car. Small consolation.

(continued on page 93)

Guidelines for Treating Childhood Insomnia

ONCE YOU UNDERSTAND these four common causes of insomnia in children, you can recognize which problems your child may have and learn how to resolve them one at a time. You need to be consistent and patient. Each problem is an acquired habit, not a sign of inadequate parenting, and can be treated over time. These problems have developed over months and need to be corrected slowly.

In the following four chapters, we present detailed guidelines for treating these four sleep disorders that often contribute to insomnia in children, but here are the basics:

STEP 1: Wean Your Child from Middle of the Night Feedings

If your baby or child is drinking (breast-feeding or bottle-feeding) through the night when she wakens, this is always the first habit you need to help her change. Your baby will not be able to sleep through the night because she is used to feeding at night, needing the calories from her food. As you wean her from drinking at night, she will naturally start to drink (breast-feed or bottle-feed) more during the day.

STEP 2: Help Your Child Fall Asleep Alone

Don't expect that as soon as your child is weaned off her nighttime feedings, she will correct the rest of her sleep problems and just sleep through the night. Even though she doesn't wake for hunger and thirst at night, she will still wake up. She needs to learn how to fall asleep in a way that will be the same both at sleep-onset (beginning of the night) and in the middle of the night without 'signaling' you for your help.

STEP 3: Set Limits So that Your Child Learns to Fall Asleep on His Own

Consider if your child has consistent, appropriate limits set on his behavior at bedtime and at night when he awakens. Some children will have difficulty settling for bed, but once asleep not waken at night. Others will have trouble accepting your attempts to change sleep associations at night, because in addition to not having learned to fall asleep alone, they also have not learned to accept limits. Whether or not your child has problems only with settling to bed at night or also with settling to bed and waking at night, recognizing the problem is the first step. You can learn how to set limits so that your child learns to stay in bed until he falls asleep on his own and when he awakens at night.

STEP 4: Adjust the Timing of Your Child's Sleep Preference

If you identify that your child has problems of sleep-onset association disorder and/or limit-setting disorder, in addition to sleeping at the wrong time, then you should try to help him with the problems listed above before tackling the timing of his sleep. For example, if he always falls asleep at 11:00 p.m., then his natural rhythms are shifted late. It is best to try the techniques described in the following chapters to teach him to fall asleep alone and to teach him new limits, but do this initially at 11:00 p.m. After you have established new patterns of falling asleep (even if it is later than you prefer), then you can gradually change the timing of his sleep.

case study: **Heather** (continued)

We assisted Martha and Gary to recognize that Heather has not one, but two problems contributing to her difficulty settling at night and waking during the night. The first is a nocturnal eating (drinking) syndrome: she is nursing all night long. The second problem is a sleep-onset association disorder: she cannot fall asleep alone without the help of a parent.

No matter what treatment strategy Martha and Gary may try, Heather will not sleep through the night until she gets used to doing this without feeding at night. Even if her parents feed her at night, rock her to sleep, and then let her 'cry it out' when she awakens, she will be very upset because she has not learned to soothe herself without drinking at night. She wakes from both hunger and thirst.

We recommended that Martha wean Heather gently off the nighttime feedings, and then teach her correct sleep associations on how to fall asleep at bedtime and through the night when she wakens without needing her parents' presence. As for their neighbor's child who cannot fall asleep unless he is taken for a car ride … that is the subject of another chapter.

Chapter 2

Nocturnal Eating (Drinking) Syndrome

MANY BABIES HAVE DIFFICULTY sleeping through the night because they are used to being nursed to sleep (breast-fed or bottle-fed) and then wake frequently at night, requiring the same feedings to return to sleep. Many babies cannot sleep through the night because of this need or habit of feeding many times at night.

Nocturnal eating (drinking) syndrome sounds like quite a mouthful (no pun intended) to describe the problem of infants and young children who eat or drink large volumes of food at times of waking during the night. In some families, a baby who wakes up frequently to breast-feed or bottle-feed at night, even at 6 months or older, is not a problem; in fact, this is a very normal sleep pattern for an infant at this age. If you do not mind the disruption to your own sleep, you can continue to get up with your baby at night, and he may eventually stretch out his sleeping periods, sleep longer, and drink less.

However, there is a good reason to try and change his hungry habits at night. The fact that he is drinking so much may also be affecting his ability to consolidate his nighttime sleep. If you try to change this pattern, you are helping him to get more restful, continuous sleep at night.

Solving nocturnal eating (drinking) problems (frequent feedings at night) is also a key to handling sleep-onset association disorder (falling asleep alone). In real life, you often cannot separate these two problems, but the first issue to resolve is always the problem of eating at night because a hungry baby cannot easily learn to sleep through the night until he is weaned from the nighttime feedings.

Did You Know?

Most Common in Infancy
Some older children and even some adults may feel the need to eat or drink during the night; however, nocturnal eating (drinking) syndrome most commonly occurs in infancy after about 6 months of age.

What Is Nocturnal Eating (Drinking) Syndrome?

Full-term, normally growing healthy infants of 6 months of age or more are able to develop the ability to sleep through the night without requiring feedings. This condition is primarily a problem of infancy and childhood.

The nighttime feedings affect your child's digestion and the release of hormones related to eating. Normally, when we sleep at night, our digestive system is resting, and the hormones related to digestion are not released. When your child is feeding frequently at night, instead of resting, his stomach is actively digesting food.

Your baby wakes up hungry because he is used to the calories or thirsty because he is used to the volume of fluids, with the result that your baby's sleep is disrupted — which, in turn, disrupts your and your partner's sleep.

WHAT THE TEXTBOOKS SAY

Nocturnal eating (drinking) syndrome is characterized by the following features:

- Your child has repeated awakenings at night and is unable to return to sleep without eating or drinking (usually drinking because this is commonly a problem in young infants).

- Your child may wake up frequently at night, commonly between three to eight times.

- After you allow your child to drink or eat the amount of food or liquid that he is used to, he is able to return to sleep rapidly.

- Your child will have excessive wetting at night, which may cause some of the wakings.

(Based on the International Classification of Sleep Disorders, 2001)

Symptoms of Nocturnal Eating (Drinking) Syndrome

If your baby has this problem, you may recognize the following symptoms. Check off any that you observe.

❑ Your baby falls asleep breast-feeding or bottle-feeding.

❑ Your baby falls asleep quickly as long as he is drinking.

❑ Once asleep, you can easily move your baby out of your arms and put him into his crib and he will stay asleep for 1 to 3 hours.

❐ Your baby wakes up frequently at night, appearing to be hungry, and cries until you feed him.

❐ Your baby falls asleep at these nighttime wakings easily as long as you let him drink.

❐ You baby's diaper needs to be changed frequently at night.

❐ Your baby drinks almost as much or more during the night as during the day.

case study: **Rosie**

Sharon and Steven brought their daughter Rosie to our sleep clinic concerned that she was not sleeping well. Rosie is a healthy, thriving 9-month-old baby girl. She falls asleep easily after nursing for 6 minutes on each breast and then can be put into the crib with no difficulty. However, about 2 hours later, she wakes up screaming and only resettles when nursed back to sleep. This pattern repeats itself every 2 to 3 hours throughout the night.

Sharon is exhausted. And although Rosie is doing well during the day because of the nighttime nursing, she is getting one-third of her daily fluid and caloric intake between midnight and 7:00 a.m.

While Sharon does not think they need help in putting Rosie to sleep at bedtime, she asked for our advice on solving the problem they have with the frequent night awakenings. They know that Rosie has problems sleeping through the night, but they do not recognize that the problem is related to how she is initially put to sleep. She has not learned to fall asleep on her own, and each time she wakes up, rather than being able to soothe herself or put herself back to sleep quickly, she becomes more awake and cries until she is fed. Sharon and Steven are exhausted, so it may be difficult to make changes in the way they put Rosie to sleep. This is the easy part of the night for them. As long as they feed her, she falls asleep very quickly.

The question became how do you help Rosie change from a baby who 'signals' or cries and needs to feed frequently at night to a baby who can soothe herself and sleeps for longer periods of time at night? We set out some guidelines for doing so . . .

(continued on page 105)

Guidelines for Treating Nighttime Eating (Drinking) Syndrome

S LOWLY WEAN YOUR child off of the food she is getting at night. Once she is used to not drinking at nighttime, she will start to drink more during the day, and the total amount of fluids and calories she is getting over 24 hours will be the same. When your child can make it through the night without drinking for a week, you can teach her to fall asleep at naptime during the day without breast-feeding or bottle-feeding.

Weaning your child of nighttime feedings can be challenging at first, but you can achieve this goal by following these steps. Check off each step as you progress.

STEP 1: Establish a Bedtime Routine

Review Part 1, Chapter 3 (Sleep Hygiene) about the importance of establishing a bedtime routine if you do not have one already in place. It may seem like your baby is too young to need a routine; however, a baby even as young as 6 months of age can benefit from a consistent, predictable, short bedtime routine that will help him understand as he develops that bedtime and sleep follow each night after the routine. Your routine with your infant or child will change as he grows, but it is an important first step in setting the stage for a smooth transition to bedtime and sleep.

STEP 2: Stop Feeding Before Your Child Is Fast Asleep

Do not change the way your child falls asleep at night until she is weaned off the nighttime feeding, except in one way. As you are weaning her from the nighttime feedings, you can continue to breast-feed or bottle-feed your child to sleep temporarily, but stop feedings before she is fast asleep and put her in the crib drowsy but slightly awake. The ultimate goal will be for your child to fall asleep without being nursed.

Note: If you are breast-feeding, follow Step 3 and 4 (Breast-feeding); if you are bottle-feeding, follow Steps 3 and 4 (Bottle-feeding) starting on page 101.

STEP 3: (Breast-Feeding): Determine Your Breast-Feeding Time Baseline

You will need to determine how much time on average your baby spends nursing at night so you can calculate the volume of fluids he is drinking. This is called baseline information. You need to know how long your baby nurses (on average) so that you can begin to decrease this time.

For three consecutive nights, gather baseline information by timing how long your baby nurses on each side each time he awakens. Following the example provided, record this information using the following blank chart. Make photocopies of the blank chart if needed.

Breast-Feeding Baseline Information Example

Take, for example, a child who breast-feeds four times a night. Nursing times are recorded for three nights in a row. Each time the baby woke up to nurse, her mother wrote down how many minutes she nursed on each breast. This baby never woke more than four times in any night, but if she had woken more often, then her mother would have continued to record the whole night. L is left side. R is right side. Time is measured in minutes.

Night	First Awakening	Second Awakening	Third Awakening	Fourth Awakening	Further Awakenings
Night # 1 Saturday	L-4 R-5	L-3 R-2	L-3 R-4	L-6 R-5	
Night # 2	L-4 R-5	L-5 R-3	L-9 R-5	No waking	
Night # 3	L-6 R-4	L-6 R-3	L-5 R-2	L-4 R-1	

Calculation

To determine where to start to wean this baby, you need to calculate the total time she nursed over these three nights.

1. First, add up all the minutes for all three nights to get the total: Total minutes per feeding on both sides = 94 minutes

2. Second, add the total number of times the baby nursed for all three nights: Total number of times the baby nursed = 11 times

3. Now, divide the total minutes by the number of times nursed to find out (on average) how long the baby nurses each time she wakes up: Average minutes per feeding 94/11 = approximately 8.5 minutes

Your Personal Breast-Feeding Baseline Information

For each time your baby wakes to feed, record the amount of time she nurses on each breast. If she only nurses on one side and falls back asleep, then record a 0 on the side that she does not nurse. L is left side. R is right side. Add columns if needed for more than five awakenings.

Night	First Awakening (minutes)	Second Awakening (minutes)	Third Awakening (minutes)	Fourth Awakening (minutes)	Further Awakenings (minutes)
Night # 1	L: R:	L: R:	L: R:	L: R:	L: R:
Night # 2	L: R:	L: R:	L: R:	L: R:	L: R:
Night # 3	L: R:	L: R:	L: R:	L: R:	L: R:

	Night #1	Night #2	Night #3
Total # Awakenings to Breast-feed			
Total minutes			

Calculation

1. Total minutes per feeding on both sides = _____ minutes
2. Total number of times the baby nursed = _____ times
3. To calculate the average minutes per feeding, divide top number (total minutes) by the bottom number (# of awakenings to nurse) = _____ minutes

STEP 4: (Breast-Feeding) Decrease Breast-Feeding Time

Each night after the first night, decrease the time nursed on each breast by about $\frac{1}{2}$ minute. Nurse the predetermined amount of time each time your baby wakes up. This may seem hard to do in the middle of the night, but keep a clock or watch handy to be able to follow this step. In the example provided, the baby's nursing time was decreased by $\frac{1}{2}$ minute in total each time she woke. In this way, the child was gently weaned from nighttime feedings over 10 to 20 days.

Schedule for Reducing Total Amount of Time Breast-Feeding on Both Sides (in minutes)

The baby in this example breast-fed for an average of 8½ minutes at baseline.

Night	First Awakening	Second Awakening	Third Awakening	Fourth Awakening	Subsequent Awakenings
1	8½	8½	8½	8½	8½
2	8	8	8	8	8
3	7½	7½	7½	7½	7½
4	7	7	7	7	7
5	6½	6½	6½	6½	6½
6	6	6	6	6	6
7	5½	5½	5½	5½	5½
8	5	5	5	5	5
9	4½	4½	4½	4½	4½
10	4	4	4	4	4
11	3½	3½	3½	3½	3½
12	3	3	3	3	3
13*	2½	2½	2½	2½	2½
14	2	2	2	2	2
15	1½	1½	1½	1½	1½
16	1	1	1	1	1
17	No nursing	No nursing	No nursing	Did not wake	Did not wake

*From night 13, when the baby is only drinking 2 minutes (even if she wakes up four times), the amount is small enough that you can just stop feeding her and do other comforting things when she wakes up for a few days until she is used to not drinking at night.

STEP 3: (Bottle-Feeding) Determine Your Bottle-feeding Amount Baseline

The method for weaning bottle-fed babies is the same as for breast-fed babies, except that you need to count the amount in ounces or milliliters your baby is drinking instead of the time spent nursing.

First, determine how much your baby is drinking at an average feeding. For three consecutive nights, measure and record how much your baby is drinking from the bottle.

Bottle-Feeding Baseline Information Example

Here is an example of an infant who was drinking between 50 and 200 milliliters each time he woke up. Amount of fluids is in milliliters (ml). Add columns if needed for more than five awakenings.

Night	First Awakening	Second Awakening	Third Awakening	Fourth Awakening	Subsequent Awakenings
Night # 1	150	200	200	Did not awaken	
Night # 2	200	150	150	150	50
Night # 3	150	200	120	180	

Calculation

To determine how to start to wean this baby, you need to calculate the total amount she consumed over these three nights.

1. First, add up all the amounts for all three nights to get the total:
   The total amount of milk this baby drank over three nights = 1900 ml
2. Second, add the total number of times the baby woke up to feed for all three nights:
   The total number of times the baby woke up to feed over three nights = 12 wakings
3. Now divide the total number of times the baby woke up to find out (on average) how much the baby nurses each time she wakes up:
   Average milliliters the baby drank per waking for the three nights is 1900/12 = approximately 160 ml

Your Personal Bottle-Feeding Baseline Information

Complete this chart for your own baby for three consecutive nights. Record the amount of fluids in milliliters.

Night	First Awakening (milliliters)	Second Awakening (milliliters)	Third Awakening (milliliters)	Fourth Awakening (milliliters)	Further Awakenings (milliliters)
Night # 1					
Night # 2					
Night # 3					

	Night #1	Night #2	Night #3
Total # Awakenings to Bottle-Feed			
Total fluids (ml)			

Calculation

1. The total amount of formula/milk your baby drank over three nights = ____ ml

2. The total number of times your baby woke up to drink over three nights = ___wakings

3. The average milliliters your baby drank per waking for the three nights is the top number (the total amount) divided by the bottom number (the number of times baby woke up) = ___ml

STEP 4: (Bottle-Feeding) Decrease Bottle-Feeding Time

Next, make a schedule to wean your baby off the nighttime feedings gradually during 10 to 20 days. Start with the baseline amount your baby drinks and decrease this amount by 15 ml each night. In our example, the baby drank on average 160 ml; therefore, every time he wakes up the first night, he will be offered 145 ml. He will not get any more formula until he falls asleep and wakes again. On the second night, he will be offered 130 ml each time he wakes up. Following this schedule, your baby will generally be weaned from nighttime feeding in 10 to 20 days.

Schedule for Reducing Total Amount of Bottle-Feeding (in milliliters)

Night	First Awakening	Second Awakening	Third Awakening	Further Awakenings
1	160	160	160	160
2	145	145	145	145
3	130	130	130	130
4	115	115	115	115
5	100	100	100	100
6	85	85	85	85
7	70	70	70	70
8	55	55	55	55
9	40	40	40	40
10	25	25	25	25
11	None	None	None	None

Tips for Weaning Babies (Breast-Fed and Bottle-Fed)

1 Be prepared for more waking during the weaning process: If your baby was waking before the weaning three to four times and now wakes five to six times, you can feed him more often, provided you continue to decrease the feedings (either the time nursing or amount in the bottle) each night. It doesn't matter that temporarily your baby may wake more and actually consume more during the night. The most important part of this step is to make sure that once you have breast-fed or bottle-fed your baby the decreased amount that you decided on, you don't give him more until the next waking. Help your baby to fall back asleep by holding, rocking, or singing to him — anything except feeding him while you are weaning him at night.

2 Don't feed your baby at each arousal more than the predetermined amount until he falls back to sleep and wakes again: Even if your child only sleeps for a shorter time, the goal of this approach is to feed him less than the night before at each awakening. In this way, you know that he is not going to be crying from hunger. He may be fussy, however, because he is used to falling asleep being entirely full and sleepy from nursing. Your child is learning slowly to fall asleep with a bit less food in his tummy and from an awakened state.

3 Be prepared to be slightly more tired during the weaning process: Try to get extra help from your partner because you will be more tired during the weaning process. Instead of just feeding your baby until he is full, and then both of you falling back to sleep, you will have to watch the time and help your baby fall back asleep by other methods. He will be somewhat fussier because he will not be as full as he likes. He may not fall asleep while he is feeding. If you are able, also plan to have extra support at home during the day. This help will allow you to rest and continue to wean your baby at night. If you are on your own, try placing the baby back in his crib and sit beside him, comforting him by singing, patting, or gently rocking him.

4 Let your baby drink/nurse as much as he wants at bedtime and during the day: While you are weaning your baby off the nighttime feedings, it is acceptable to let him nurse as long as he wants or bottle-feed as much fluid as he wants when he falls asleep at bedtime and at naps. In addition to letting him drink as much as he wants, you can also try putting him in his crib drowsy but slightly awake, rather than falling asleep on the breast or bottle. Offer him more when he is awake. You do not want to create too much stress for yourself or for your baby. Take one step at a time. The first step is to wean him off the nighttime feedings.

5 If bottle-feeding, make up the bottles in the evening with the correct amount: You can make some extra bottles since initially your baby may wake up more often. Give him the same amount each time, but do not worry if he wakes up a few more times. As he is weaned off breast milk or formula, he may resume his previous waking schedule, but if not, you are going to teach him to settle himself when he wakes in the next chapter.

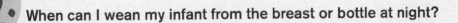

Q. **When can I wean my infant from the breast or bottle at night?**

A. Once your baby is over 6 months old, and if he is healthy and thriving, talk to your health-care provider about weaning him off nighttime feedings. At this age, babies can tolerate larger amounts of milk and can be fed less frequently, eating more during the day or early evening. Some infants may still need a midnight feeding, but at 9 months of age, 70% to 80% of infants sleep through the night without food.

Q. **Will watering down formula or milk help wean my child off frequent nighttime feedings?**

A. You may be told to give your baby watered-down formula or just substitute water to help your baby get used to fewer calories and eventually less fluid. This practice is not recommended. Continuing with the full-strength formula will be easier on your baby. He will still be slowly weaned off the nighttime feeding, but he will continue to have sufficient calories so that the weaning process will be gentler.

case study: **Rosie** (continued)

Rosie successfully learned to get through the night without nursing. She now has a consistent sleep routine in her bedroom for 5 to 10 minutes at naptime and bedtime. This consists of a song and cuddling by her mother or father. Then she is nursed until she is drowsy but awake and placed into her crib.

Rosie still wakes at night because she has not learned to soothe herself to sleep, but she drinks and eats more during the day. When she wakens, her father gets up with her and rocks her until she falls back asleep. This is acceptable for the short term. Her parents are now ready to teach Rosie to fall asleep on her own from a waking state without them soothing her or needing to be with her.

Chapter 3

Sleep-Onset Association Disorder

SLEEP ASSOCIATIONS ARE the conditions present when we fall asleep. Infants, like all of us, fall asleep in a certain way and have cycles of sleep with repeated brief episodes of arousal. This is a normal sleep pattern. These associations become problematic when your infant or child cannot soothe himself back to sleep at night and needs you or your partner to recreate the same conditions he had while falling asleep the first time in order to do so. Not all sleep associations are problematic — some healthy associations may improve the quality and quantity of your child's sleep.

Did You Know?

Next Step
The next step in treating childhood insomnia is to teach your baby to fall asleep, not only without being breast-fed or bottle-fed, but also without disruptive sleep associations, such as excessive rocking, cuddling, even being driven around town in a car, or any other activity that he needs you for. In other words, you want your baby to learn how to soothe himself to sleep.

What Is Sleep-Onset Association Disorder?

We all have our own sleep associations. For example, you may prefer to sleep on the left side of the bed, with the hall light on, and two pillows. If you have these same conditions every night, you are able to fall asleep easily, and during your brief arousals at night, you are comforted at a subconscious level by seeing that the same associations are present. You fall back asleep easily, not even being aware of waking at night.

However, if you find yourself sleeping in a hotel room, and you only have one pillow, and the light and room conditions are different from what you are used to, you may not have quite as restful a sleep. In the morning, you may not be aware of the brief episodes of arousal you had the previous night. If you were to be videotaped sleeping in this different environment, your arousals would be slightly longer as you looked around the room to try to understand what was different about your environment and, consequently, in the morning you may not feel as rested as if you had slept at home.

This also applies to your baby. If your baby routinely falls asleep while you are nursing or rocking him, he may need the same conditions re-created every time when he wakes up. While these brief wakings are normal through the night, your baby needs to learn to fall back asleep without requiring your assistance.

Don't worry if you use these techniques to help your young infant to fall asleep. Until about 6 months of age, some newborns and babies can fall asleep on their own, but others need to be rocked or nursed to sleep. These associations can be problematic when they become a habit for your older infant, toddler, or child who has not learned to settle to sleep on his own.

WHAT THE TEXTBOOKS SAY

Sleep-onset association disorder is characterized by the following features:

- Your child is unable to fall asleep at naptime or bedtime unless a certain object or set of circumstances is present.

- When these conditions are present, your child has a normal sleep pattern; however, when the conditions are not present, transitions to sleep at bedtime and after nighttime wakings are delayed.

- Although it may seem like the number of times that your child wakens at night is excessive, it is probably part of a normal sleep pattern. This becomes a problem when your child cannot settle himself back to sleep on his own.

- When you recreate the required conditions (for example, rocking, cuddling, singing, or nursing), then your child falls back to sleep quickly.

- The sleep-onset association conditions usually require participation by you, your partner, or your child's caregiver.

- This problem is mainly a childhood sleep problem.

(Based on the International Classification of Sleep Disorders, 2001)

Correct or Adaptive Sleep Associations

The conditions that do not require the presence of a parent or other caregiver at the time of falling asleep or at the time of night wakings are called correct sleep associations. The words adaptive, positive, or good can also be used for these types of associations with sleep. A child with correct sleep associations can fall asleep from the awake state on his own and with the bedroom environment (light level, noise level) unchanged from the time he goes to sleep until the time he wakes up in the morning.

Correct Associations

Correct sleep associations are present when we fall asleep and do not change during the night. For a baby, this could include:

- Falling asleep consistently in the same crib or bassinet
- Falling asleep in the same room each night
- Falling asleep with a low level of light or night-light on all night
- Falling asleep in a quiet room
- Falling asleep with a special blanket — or in an older child, with a toy or stuffed animal

Incorrect or Problematic Sleep Associations

Incorrect sleep associations require parental presence at times of falling asleep or night waking. Incorrect sleep associations are objects, environmental factors, or people who are present when your child falls asleep, but absent when he has natural arousals through the night and have to be recreated for him to fall back asleep.

To help their children get to sleep, parents may unknowingly establish bad habits, which become problematic associations. You may not know the importance of adaptive and problematic sleep associations and how they can disrupt your child's sleep.

Incorrect Associations

These associations are not problematic for a baby under 4 to 6 months of age. At this early age, you should help your baby fall asleep because some young babies are not able to make the transition from awake to sleep.

- Falling asleep outside of the bedroom and being moved into bed once your child is sleeping
- Falling asleep with another person in the bed (it may be a parent, sibling, or other family member); it is only a problem if the person the child falls asleep with moves once the child is sleeping
- Falling asleep with rocking, patting, rubbing, or massaging
- Falling asleep with singing or playing music
- Falling asleep with the radio or television on
- Falling asleep while driving in the car
- Falling asleep while walking in the stroller
- Falling asleep with a bottle
- Falling asleep using a pacifier

Did You Know?

Constant Environment
You can help your baby fall asleep at bedtime and fall back asleep when he wakes through the night by providing a constant sleep environment. Your baby will learn to associate his own crib in a quiet, dimly lit room as cues to fall asleep.

Did You Know?

Pacifier Advice
The pacifier is listed as an incorrect sleep association because your baby or child may use it to fall asleep and can't put it back in his own mouth when he wakens. However, using a pacifier is one of the risk factors thought to be associated with a decreased incidence of SIDS. Once your child is more than 1 year old and the risk of SIDS is not a concern, you should definitely consider the pacifier as a cause of incorrect sleep associations and try to eliminate it from the sleep routine for your child.

Symptoms of Sleep-Onset Association Disorder

Check your baby for the following common symptoms of sleep-onset association disorder. In infants, the disorder may spontaneously resolve itself at any time. Often, however, symptoms persist until age 3 or 4 years old when nursing, sucking on bottles or pacifiers, rocking, and holding decrease markedly. Untreated, the course is variable.

- Your child falls asleep easily, often in minutes as long as you rock, nurse, drive in the car, give him his pacifier, or create other soothing associations.

- Your child is unable to fall asleep easily if you put him to bed awake and do not do the things he is used to.

- Once asleep, you can move your child to bed, without waking him.

- When he wakes up at night (which happens up to eight times a night), you can easily get him back to sleep by doing the same things you did to get him to fall asleep at bedtime.

- In the morning, your child appears well rested, but you are very tired from waking up often at night. This will be the case in general. If you recreate the conditions that allowed your child to fall asleep quickly at bedtime, his sleep will only be disrupted minimally.

Sleep-Onset Association Disorder in Toddlers

When a toddler or preschooler has sleep-onset association disorder, she may resist going to bed or go to bed easily only if she has particular conditions at bedtime (usually having at least one of her parents present), but she has difficulty maintaining sleep through the night. While this a common type of sleep disturbance in a toddler, you should take it seriously because research studies show that if a young child doesn't sleep well, she may continue to have this problem for many years.

Family Dynamics

If you and your partner are going to make behavioral changes with your child, you need to agree on the treatment option and be consistent with your approach. You need to consider your own cultural and family background, which affects your beliefs and attitudes as a parent, and talk about the differences you may have with your partner. Sometimes the child's apparent sleep problem masks an underlying marital problem. These family dynamics need to be evaluated and resolved.

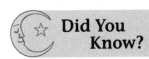

Did You Know?

Medical Vs. Behavioral Problems
If your child has a significant medical problem that interferes with her sleep, she will not be able to sleep under any circumstance. If your child has a problem related to behavior, she will be able to sleep in some settings. For example, she may sleep when she is in bed all night with someone, when she is at her grandparents' home and sleeps in their bed, or when you are traveling and sharing a room with her.

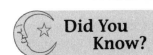

Did You Know?

Spontaneous Waking
Preschoolers and school-age children (until the teenage years) should wake up spontaneously in the morning without much help from their parents. If your child has much difficulty waking in the morning, this is a sign that he is not getting enough sleep, most likely from a bedtime that is too late or from the night waking disturbing his sleep.

SLEEP-ONSET ASSOCIATION QUESTIONNAIRE

These questions may help you determine if your toddler has a sleep-onset association disorder. Check off questions that apply to your child.

☐ Can your child sleep easily when he has the proper circumstances? For example, can he fall asleep only if he has you lying beside him, or if he has his favorite music playing, or if you take him for a drive in the car?

☐ Does your child wake up several times at night?

☐ When your child wakes up at night, does he fall back to sleep easily when you go to him and recreate the same conditions in which he fell asleep at bedtime?

☐ Are there any nights when your child sleeps through the night – for example, if you are traveling and sleeping with your child in the same room?

case study: **Andrew**

When Andrew came to our sleep clinic, his parents, Emma and Matthew, were at their wits' end. Andrew is their first and only child, a bright, rambunctious 2½-year-old, who is fairly easy-going.

However, his nursery school teacher reports that he seems tired in the morning and sometimes he initiates fights for no apparent reason with his peers. At night, he successfully keeps his father out of the bedroom. Andrew will only fall asleep in his parents' bedroom with his mother lying beside him, while touching his mother's ear, which allows him to fall asleep easily.

Emma and Matthew are not happy with this arrangement. After falling asleep, they gently move Andrew to his own bedroom. If they wait just the right amount of time to move him, he will sleep soundly even while being carried. He consistently wakes up three to four times through the night, gets out of his bed, and 'kicks' his father out of the parental bed so he can get back in to fall asleep with his mother again. During the daytime, Andrew does not have a nap, but will often fall asleep when in the car or watching television.

Emma and Matthew thought the problem could be resolved by making Andrew's bedroom more comfortable. Because he seemed to prefer the bigger bed in his parents' room, they replaced his bed with a double bed in his own bedroom. None of this helped, though his father is now more comfortable when he goes to sleep in Andrew's room.

We diagnosed Andrew with sleep-onset association disorder and recommended a number of treatment options....

(continued on page 124)

Guidelines for Treating Infants with Sleep-Onset Association Disorder

THE WAY TO TEACH your baby to sleep more continuously and not require your assistance at night is to help him learn to fall asleep on his own. You want to change the associations he has with falling asleep from those that need your presence to those that will be present when he is alone in his crib or bed. Then, he will learn to sleep longer without needing you frequently at night.

Your child will still briefly wake at night, but instead of 'signaling' or crying excessively until you come and help him to fall asleep by doing the same thing you did at bedtime, he will learn to quietly soothe himself and fall back asleep without you. This will be good for both of you. You and your baby will each get more sleep.

However, your baby won't be able to learn to soothe himself in the middle of the night until he learns to do this at bedtime. That is why it is not a good idea to help your baby fall asleep at night at bedtime and then just let him 'cry it out' at night. If he can't fall asleep at bedtime on his own, you can't expect him to be able to do this when he wakes up in the middle of the night. If you rock him to sleep at bedtime, and then ignore him when he wakes up later, you are expecting him to be able to soothe himself in the middle of the night when he hasn't learned how to do this.

Your baby must learn to fall asleep by himself without needing you to be present. In order to do this, you need to slowly remove the incorrect sleep associations and replace them with correct or positive associations. The goal is to change his sleep habits gradually so that he can be in his crib drowsy or awake and fall asleep on his own.

STEP 1: Wean from Nighttime Feeding

The first step to improving sleep is to wean your baby off of his nighttime feedings if he breast-feeds or bottle-feeds at night. You do this by calculating how much he drinks on an average night and slowly decreasing the amount until he is able to get through the night without drinking. As you are weaning him off his nighttime feedings, you increase other comforting measures, such as rocking, singing, and cuddling, to help him fall asleep without drinking. While doing this, you change slightly how you put him to sleep at bedtime and naptimes. You stop feeding him before he is entirely full and put him in the crib, drowsy, but slightly awake. See Part 3, Chapter 2, "Nocturnal Eating (Drinking) Syndrome," for additional guidelines.

STEP 2: Sleep in a Comfortable Environment

The room where your baby sleeps should be quiet and dark, with a night-light if required. If there is a night-light on at night, it should stay on the same level all night. You want the environment of the room to be the same when your baby falls asleep as when he wakes up during the night.

STEP 3: Start at Naptime

Once your baby can get through the night without feeding, then the next step is to teach him to fall asleep alone without any parental intervention. Try teaching him to fall asleep alone during the day at naptime if possible. This may be easier for you because you are not so tired. Do this at only one naptime — at bedtime and at nighttime, you can continue to comfort him using the associations you have established. Do not go back to feeding him when he is falling asleep, though.

If you are working during the day, you can choose to start this sleep training on the weekend and have your caregiver continue during the week — or just reverse the steps and teach your baby to fall asleep at nighttime first, and then have your caregiver use the same techniques during the day for naps. The more consistent you are, having your partner, other family members, and caregivers use the same sleep training techniques, the easier it will be to improve your baby's sleep habits.

STEP 4: Remove Incorrect Sleep-Onset Associations

Some children have developed not one, but multiple sleep associations. If your child has multiple associations — for example, you walk with him in the living room with lights and the television on until he falls asleep — you need to remove these interventions one at a time. You should be consistent and follow these steps both at naptime and at bedtime.

Sample Sleep-Onset Association Correction Routine

Here is an 11-day routine to correct problematic sleep-onset associations one at a time:

Day 1 to 3: Select one of your child's sleep associations — in this case, falling asleep with the television on in the living room. Turn off the television. Instead of walking with your child in the living room, move to the room where he sleeps (your room or his own) with the lights dimmed until he falls asleep. In this first step, he will be learning to associate sleep with a quiet, darkened room.

Day 4 to 6: Next, teach your child to fall asleep in his crib or bed, not in your arms. In the room where your baby sleeps, put him into his crib, drowsy but awake, and sit beside him with physical contact, rubbing or patting him, for example, in his bed. In this step, he will be learning to associate sleep with his own crib, but you are still beside him for comfort. You have removed one problematic association, which is holding him and rocking him to sleep.

Day 7 to 10: Now, teach your child to fall asleep with you present, but not in contact. Follow the same routine as the previous day, but now when you put your baby in the crib, sit beside him without any constant physical contact, such as rubbing, rocking, or patting him in the crib. You can sit beside him and occasionally touch him to soothe him. Do not sing to him or do other actions that he will enjoy and that may encourage him to stay awake rather than to go to sleep.

7-Day Schedule for Sleeping Alone

When you follow this schedule, your interactions with your baby should be brief. When you go to him, pat him gently and quickly in the crib, calmly say some words, such as "good night," then leave the room quickly.

Do not pick him up and hug and cuddle him. This is called positive reinforcement. The more pleasant you make the contact with him, the more he will cry when you leave. Some babies who are very determined (later in life this is a good trait) will cry for hours the first few nights. However, most babies will have stopped fussing and fallen asleep after the first few days of following a consistent schedule.

In this example, the time is increased each time your baby wakens until he wakens four times in one night. If your baby wakens more than four times, continue to wait the same minutes as you did at the fourth waking before re-entering his room.

Day	Time to wait at first waking	Time to wait at second waking	Time to wait at third waking	Time to wait at fourth waking	Subsequent wakings
Day 1	2 minutes	4 minutes	6 minutes	8 minutes	8 minutes
Day 2	4 minutes	6 minutes	8 minutes	10 minutes	10 minutes
Day 3	6 minutes	8 minutes	10 minutes	12 minutes	12 minutes
Day 4	8 minutes	10 minutes	12 minutes	14 minutes	14 minutes
Day 5	10 minutes	12 minutes	14 minutes	16 minutes	16 minutes
Day 6	12 minutes	14 minutes	16 minutes	18 minutes	18 minutes
Day 7	14 minutes	16 minutes	18 minutes	20 minutes	20 minutes

Day 11: By now, your baby has learned that you are gradually withdrawing your contact in a gentle way as he falls asleep. Now, it is time to follow your bedtime routine by putting your baby in his crib and leaving the room.

Onwards: If he is older than 9 months, be prepared for your baby to be upset when you get to Day 11 because at this age he will have developed 'object permanency', which means he knows the difference between your presence and absence. After his feeding and bedtime routine, you put him into the crib. After the 'good night' routine, you leave the room where he cannot hear or see you. Then, you can reenter the room at periodic intervals to reassure him that you haven't abandoned him — and to reassure yourself that your baby is fine.

STEP 5: Set a Schedule for Sleeping Alone

To continue to support your baby so that he does not feel you are abandoning him and, at the same time, to teach him to be able to fall asleep alone, you can use the following schedule. This schedule describes a method to check on your baby without reinforcing his crying until he learns to fall asleep alone.

Scheduling Tips

1 **Be flexible:** The time you wait does not matter, just that you follow a consistent schedule increasing the time you wait each night. Although the schedule suggests waiting 2 minutes and then adding 2 minutes to each subsequent wait time, this is not a rule. There is no scientific evidence for the amount of time needed for the waits between checking your baby. The only strategy that is important in this type of gentle training is that you wait longer each time before you go to your baby.

2 **Increase waiting time:** If you go to see your baby every 2 minutes, he will quickly realize that if he cries for 2 minutes, he is going to see you soon. If you keep increasing the time, he will not be able to predict when you are coming and will learn to fall asleep on his own.

Therefore, if you want to change the time that you wait, you can start with 5 minutes, 1 minute, 30 seconds or any other time you choose. The schedule will work provided you continue to increase the time that you wait. If your baby wakes up more than five to six times at night, you can continue to go in at set intervals for any further times without the increase. However most babies will fall asleep long before this if you follow these suggestions.

3 **Try using a transitional object:** A special object, such as a blanket or, for an older child, a stuffed animal may help your child to fall asleep initially and when he wakes at night. This transitional object can be used when sleeping away from home.

4 **Consider combining this gentle approach with the 'cold-turkey' approach:** When you are following this schedule, you may start to hear your baby quieting down, but when you go into the room, his crying intensifies when he sees you. This is a good time to try the 'cold turkey' approach by waiting outside his room longer than in the schedule and listening without letting your baby see you to determine if he is going to settle on his own. You can use a combination of these approaches. We do not advocate letting a baby cry for long periods of time.

5 **Use a schedule at naptime to start:** Once your baby has fallen asleep by himself at naptime, then you can call this a success, and even if he wakes up in 15 minutes or only has a short nap, you can do any nurturing thing he likes (except feed him) to get him back to sleep for the rest of his nap. This can include using rocking, singing, or any other comforting activity. The goal of this step is to teach him to fall asleep from being awake and alone. Congratulate yourself when you reach this goal.

STEP 6: Respond Properly to Your Baby

Once your baby can fall asleep alone and is not drinking anything at night, he will probably stop needing you to help him fall back asleep when he has the natural brief wakings that we all have at night. Your child will have learned to be a 'self-soother'. However, he may still need you from time to time.

1 If your child wakes at night and still needs you, make this encounter brief and loving. Do not reinforce these wakings by picking him up, comforting him, and encouraging him to want to interact with you at night.

2 In the same way you taught him to fall asleep at night, you should go to him at increasing time intervals, stay with him briefly, and then leave the room. The goal is to reassure him that you have not abandoned him and to reassure yourself that he is safe, warm, and comfortable. You can pat his back or tummy, depending on how he is lying, speak in quiet soothing words, and then say "good night" and leave the room. If he is standing in the crib, as long as he cannot climb out of the crib, you can help him lie down, or just tell him that it is nighttime and leave the room.

3 Try not to turn on the lights. Don't play any music.

4 You can listen for his noises from outside the room, but once you have left the room, don't let him see or hear you. In this way, he is learning to go back to sleep on his own when he wakes up at night.

Guidelines for Treating Toddlers with Sleep-Onset Association Disorder

TO CHANGE PROBLEMATIC sleep associations to healthy sleep associations, we recommend a behavior treatment called graduated extinction, which means that you are slowly teaching your toddler or older child to fall asleep on his own by minimizing your interactions with her at the time of sleep onset. The research shows that these techniques are safe and very effective in improving sleep in infants and children.

STEP 1: Establish a Bedtime and Naptime Routine and Schedule

Before beginning to correct the actual problem of incorrect sleep associations, you need to establish a bedtime and naptime routine and schedule. This will tell your child at each nap and at bedtime that it is time to go to sleep. The routine will be predictable. Toddlers like routines and predictability. The bedtime routine can be practiced for 1 week before making any other changes in your child's sleep habits. See Part 1, Chapter 3, "Sleep Hygiene," for more information on establishing a bedtime routine.

STEP 2: Determine Your Child's Sleep-Onset Associations

Make a list of all the sleep associations your child has when going to sleep at bedtime and at nighttime arousals. Separate these into correct (adaptive) and incorrect (maladaptive) associations.

My Child's Sleep-Onset Association List

List your child's sleep associations and evaluate them as correct or incorrect by checking the appropriate column.

Sleep Association	Correct/Adaptive	Incorrect/Maladaptive

STEP 3: Change Maladaptive Sleep Associations

Change the maladaptive associations, one at a time. The behavior change should be consistent and gentle. Both parents should be in agreement with this effort to change their child's sleep habits and share the same positive, supportive, non-punitive approach.

① Be prepared for some disruption and upset times in this part of the sleep training. Your child may not fully understand why you are changing his routine and will be resistant to this change. He does not see the reason to change things and enjoys the status quo. He is not used to being the one who is not in charge.

② Be consistent, calm, and confident of your actions to teach him to fall asleep alone. Discuss this change with your child, but keep the discussion brief. Let him know that, in the end, he will feel better, sleep better, develop healthy sleep habits, and his family will also be happier.

③ Remember that your child is not causing difficulties at night because he is a bad or a spoiled child. The way that he falls asleep is simply a habit, but it is not currently a good habit. You are teaching him better, healthier sleep habits. You are going to do everything slowly, supporting your child. There is no punishment involved, even though he may show poor behavior initially when you start to make changes.

STEP 4: Reduce Parental Associations

The common problem of toddlers and children needing to sleep with their mother (or sometimes their father) to fall asleep can be treated using behavioral strategies. By this time, your child is out of the crib, so you need to create a 'crib-like barrier' to teach him to stay in his own bed at night when he is falling asleep.

You can try using two child gates at his door, one on top of the other so he can't climb over. Or you can intermittently close his door when he is not cooperating with the changes so that he cannot get out of the room by himself.

A more effective strategy may be to use graduated extinction behavior treatments to teach your child to fall asleep without his mother. Graduated extinction behavior treatment sounds like you are going to be using sophisticated therapy with your child. Actually, it is quite simple — you are changing a behavior in your child by withdrawing your involvement with him while he falls asleep. One option is called a chair-sitting strategy, while another is known as timed-waiting or intermittent door closing.

Chair-Sitting Strategy

This treatment involves you or your partner sitting in a chair and slowly moving away from your child while he is in his bed until you are out of the bedroom and he can no longer see you. This is done in a progressive way by moving the chair in increments every night farther away from your child.

Chair-Sitting Steps

1. Put a chair right beside your child's bed, and let your child touch you (if he is used to being in physical contact with you) until he falls asleep. Do not lie in bed.
2. Put the chair right beside the bed, but stop physical contact with your child.
3. Put the chair right beside the bed, but turn it away from your child so there is no eye contact. Do not talk to your child while he is falling asleep.
4. Move the chair in increments away from the side of the bed every night. The amount that you move it will depend on the size of the room. Move it every night a little farther, and continue to have it facing away from your child so that there is no verbal or eye contact.
5. Continue moving the chair until it is in the hall and your child can no longer hear or see you as he is falling asleep.

If your child is a little older, you can involve him more in this routine, giving him some control during the day of the changes that you are making at night. During the day, you can have him help you mark the floor where the chair will be that night. You can make a chart and post it showing the movement of the chair and how long it will take to move out of the room. You can have a reward system with stickers for his cooperation with this behavioral change.

When you are teaching your child to fall asleep at bedtime, you should leave once he is asleep. If your child wakes up in the middle of the night, you can do anything necessary to get everyone back to bed quickly. This can include bringing him into bed with you or lying down with him. The goal at this stage is simply to work on changing one sleep habit — teaching him to fall asleep on his own.

Timed-Waiting Strategy

In this method of changing behavior, the goal is for your child to be in bed alone at night while falling asleep. Some families prefer to just go right to this timed-waiting method and not use the chair-sitting routine, especially if your child is not cooperating with the chair-sitting strategy.

Using this timed-waiting method, you are gradually withdrawing from your child in the room for progressively longer intervals. You are not abandoning your child, leaving him upset in his room until he falls asleep. You are going to check on your child at progressively longer time intervals. In this way, you are reassured that he is safe, and he is reassured that he is not abandoned. This is very similar to teaching an infant to fall asleep. The only difference is that there is no crib to enforce 'controls' on your preschooler, so you need to ensure he stays in his room by temporarily closing his bedroom door to ensure cooperation.

Each time you go in to check on your child, you should be brief, calm, and patient. You are just checking on him, so a quick visit (less than 1 minute) is all you need to reiterate, "It is time to go to bed, you are fine, good night." If you make it a positive interaction, you may encourage him to continue to stay awake in order to see you. If you have a negative interaction, your child may still prefer to see you in any capacity, even tired and unhappy with him. Remember that he is not having trouble falling asleep because he is naughty; he has just learned poor sleeping habits and needs to learn good habits.

Timed-Waiting Steps

1. After your bedtime routine, say "good night" and leave your child awake and in his room.

2. You don't need to close the door unless your child will not stay in his room. If he will stay in his room, then just leave the room where he cannot see or hear you.

3. If he does not stay in his room, give your child a choice. You can say something calmly, such as "If you stay in the room, I'll leave the door open. If you come out of the room, I'll close and hold the door."

4. If your child comes out of his bedroom, calmly place him back in bed, close his door, and wait while he stays in his room. Do not speak to him while waiting.

5. Wait progressively longer intervals, leaving him in his room for longer time periods. In between each time, open the door and go back into the room. When you do this, you give your child the choice again: "If you stay in the room, I'll leave the door open. If you come out of the room, then I'll close the door."

6. When you close the door, hold it closed (if necessary) without talking to your child from behind the closed door. Again, even the sound of your calm or angry voice behind the door is more pleasant for your child than being in the room without you.

7. If you are worried that your child is going to harm himself in his room (for example, he becomes so angry that he pulls down the bedside lamp), be sure to make the room very safe by removing objects that he could be harmful.

8. Then establish a graduated schedule you'll be following for this intermittent door-closing strategy.

Graduated Schedule for Timed-Waiting Intermittent Door Closing (in minutes)

If your child wakes up more than four times, continue each time with the same time as in the fourth wait.

Night	First Wait	Second Wait	Third Wait	Fourth Wait	Subsequent Wait
Night # 1	2	4	6	8	8
Night # 2	4	6	8	10	10
Night # 3	6	8	10	12	12
Night # 4	8	10	12	14	14
Night # 5	10	12	14	16	16
Night # 6	12	14	16	18	18
Night # 7	14	16	18	20	20

⑨ If the time is up and your child is still upset, check on him, no matter what state he is in. Calmly open the door, help him back into his bed (if he will cooperate), and say "good night" again. Then leave the room. If he refuses to get into bed and even if he is in the middle of a temper tantrum, just say some calming words and leave the room with the door open or shut, depending on if he will stay in the room or not. For the first few nights, your child may fall asleep right on the floor in front of the door; however, after a few nights, when he realizes that this will not change your resolve to improve his sleep habits, he will start to go to bed to fall asleep.

Once your child falls asleep at bedtime without you in the room, and with only correct sleep associations, any problems with falling back to sleep after night awakenings will likely resolve on their own or with little intervention. If your child does wake at night, you can go back to the chair-sitting or timed-waiting routine if needed.

Tips for Reducing Parental Associations

1. **Share responsibility:** With your partner, alternate nights putting your child to bed. However, you should only do this if you both agree on being calm and consistent so that your child knows what to expect (the same method) from both parents. If one parent gets frustrated easily and is more prone to negative interactions, then the other parent should take care of teaching correct sleep habits. Once your child learns to cooperate and fall asleep alone, then both parents alternately share the pleasure of putting your child to bed at night.

2. **Limit your expectations and be persistent:** You may feel exhausted and frustrated if it takes 2 hours to get your child to fall asleep and then he wakes up in 1 hour wanting to get back into your bed. Remember, the only goal at this time is to teach your child to fall asleep alone without you present. You are not necessarily expecting him to sleep through the night. You are not expected to be able to carry out this type of behavior management all night long. That would be too exhausting for anyone.

3. **Be flexible:** Once your child falls asleep having carried out these strategies, whenever he wakes up, do any nurturing thing you need to (including the old habits of bringing him back into your bed) so that everyone gets some sleep. The next night, just work on falling asleep again. Once he learns to fall asleep with the correct associations, he will start to self-soothe and put himself back to sleep without you. If he does not, you can do this same behavior management for night awakenings.

FREQUENTLY ASKED QUESTIONS

Q *These chair-sitting and timed-waiting methods don't seem to work for our child. In fact, they seem to make the problem worse. What should we do?*

A This is a common question frustrated parents ask their doctor. You may be tempted to abandon the routine, but stick with it. It is a normal behavior for your child to become more upset before things improve. Your child would prefer not to change. His resistance is an attempt to convince you to go back to the behavior that he prefers. But remember that you are changing a problematic sleep habit so that everyone in your family will enjoy better sleep.

continued on next page

Q *The chair-sitting method seemed to be working until I got too far away from my child, and then he wanted me to start over again and sit close enough to him that I could touch him while he falls asleep. What should I do?*

A You may need to combine the two methods, the chair-sitting and the timed-waiting routines. If you get to the point where you have moved the chair away from the bed, rather than move it closer (which would be like starting again), you can tell your child that if he cooperates with the placement of the chair, you will stay in the chair until he falls asleep. However, if he gets out of bed or does not cooperate in any way, calmly leave the room and use the timed-waiting routine, where you close the door for progressively longer times until your child either falls asleep or agrees that you can sit in the chair where you have left it.

Q *I've tried these methods before and they didn't work for my child. What else can I try?*

A Sometimes, these methods do not work, often because the family was not consistent and persistent in continuing to make changes in a gradual, supportive way. Often parents try to make changes for a few nights or even a week, but then they give up due to frustration or exhaustion. If this sounds familiar, it may be helpful to talk to your doctor about the problem with your child's sleep so that he can offer you support while you are carrying out these behavioral changes. Other problems that may be interfering with being able to carry out these changes include difficulties in your home, in your marriage, or in your (or your partner's) own mental health. If you are concerned that these problems are interfering with your ability to carry out a behavior program to improve your child's sleep, talk to your doctor about these issues.

Q *My child is quite anxious about most things, especially change. These treatments only seem to increase his anxiety. What should we do?*

A For some children, these methods do not work, especially if they have difficulty with anxiety and separating from you, both during the day and at bedtime. These methods may cause greater anxiety when your child feels separated from you. If this is the case with your child, be sure to consult with your doctor. See Part 3, Chapter 8, "Nightmares and Nighttime Anxiety," for more information.

Q *What should we do if our child stays in his room, but he plays in bed for hours and won't go to sleep?*

A You cannot make anyone fall asleep. You do not want to put your child to bed and do this sleep training when he is not ready to fall asleep. Try starting the bedtime routine at a time when your child is tired, and do this training when he would naturally be falling asleep. Once you get him to fall asleep, you can gradually move his bedtime back to a more desirable bedtime. Also see Part 3, Chapter 5, "Circadian Rhythm Sleep Disorders," for more information on delayed sleep phase preference.

Q *What do I do if my child sleeps in a bedroom with a sibling?*

A Helping your child to change his sleeping habits may upset the sleep of other family members, especially if he sleeps with siblings in the same room or bed. If this is the case, you will need to move the sibling to another room, temporarily.

Q *We live in an apartment and I think that our neighbors will hear the noise and call the police if I try to use these suggestions?*

A If you are worried that your child's fussing will bother your neighbors, you can still use these strategies. Explain to your neighbors ahead of time what you will be doing and that you will not be punishing your child. Let them know that they may hear your child fussing and crying when he has new limits set on his sleep behavior at night. You can assure your neighbor that this will be a temporary situation because, if you are consistent with these techniques, your child will soon learn to stay in bed at night and fall asleep quietly.

Q *What do we do when we are traveling and sleeping together in one room?*

A If you are traveling, staying at someone's home or in a hotel, it is likely you are going to have different sleeping arrangements, together in one room or sharing rooms. Continue as much as possible with the schedule. Keep the bedtime routine as similar as possible to the home routine. However, this is not the time to be instilling better sleep habits. Do whatever you need to in order to get everyone to sleep (in that way you will be invited back if you are staying in someone's home) and then when you get home, go back to the chair-sitting or timed-waiting approach where you had left off.

Q *What do I do if my child gets sick?*

A You should feel no pressure to teach your child to fall asleep quickly at any one time. If you have started any part of this training with an infant, whether it is weaning off fluids at night or teaching your baby to fall asleep at night, you should temporarily abandon this training if he becomes ill and use all your nurturing strategies to help him to sleep at night until he has recovered. If your infant develops a fever, stomach virus, or other illness, he may need more fluids. This is not the time to be restricting fluids or causing your baby any additional stress. When he has recovered, you can start from where you began and continue to help your baby learn to sleep through the night.

If your child is 3 or 4 years of age, he has had the same sleep habits for several years. When he is ill or under extraordinary stress (for example, from a death in the family, or from getting ready to go to kindergarten), be flexible. At times of sickness or stress, use whatever method you used in the past to get everyone in the family to sleep. When the crisis or sickness is passed, start the chair-sitting or timed-waiting strategies again. However, even in times of illness or stress, it is still beneficial to have a sleep-wake schedule and a bedtime routine. This structure will give your child comfort in his life that will help him to cope with extra stress.

case study: **Andrew** (continued)

After some consideration, Andrew's parents were able to list his problematic sleep associations:

- He falls asleep in our room
- He holds his mother's ear while falling asleep
- He needs his mother with him lying down in bed while falling asleep
- He has a music box turned on while falling asleep
- He has the bedroom light on so his mother can read while he falls asleep

With his parents, we established the three-part goal of having Andrew go to bed in his own room at bedtime, fall asleep on his own, and learn to sleep through the night in his own bedroom without requiring any parental assistance. To help them achieve this goal, we broke it down into several stages.

To enable Andrew to fall asleep in his own bedroom, even if he has to have his mother or father present while falling asleep, his parents established a consistent bedtime routine with Andrew in his own bedroom. They changed the place where Andrew falls asleep from their bedroom to his own bedroom. Temporarily, Emma lies down at bedtime and occasionally sleeps with Andrew in his room. The goal is one change at a time.

We emphasized that we are not trying to improve the whole night, just to teach Andrew that he can fall asleep in his own room. When Andrew wakes at night, his mother can do any other comforting things to get him (and herself) back to sleep.

We also stressed how important it was for Andrew to accept his father, Matthew, settling him at night. While teaching Andrew to fall asleep in his room, Matthew and Emma alternated lying down with him. This is ideal. However, if Andrew only accepts his mother at bedtime, this long-standing problem can be resolved at a later stage, and, temporarily, Emma alone can teach Andrew to fall asleep at bedtime.

The next step we recommended was to wean Andrew off his incorrect or maladaptive sleep associations. The easiest things to change were turning off the music and the light, so for 3 nights they kept a night-light on dimly at the same level of light as when he fell asleep. After 3 days, Andrew was falling asleep in a darkened, quiet environment.

These changes in Andrew's sleep associations were not all that stressful. His mother and father were still with him in his room when he was falling asleep. Removing themselves from the room was more difficult for Emma and Matthew. However, following our guidelines for the chair-sitting routine, they were able to change this habit. Andrew now goes to sleep most nights by himself, without any maladaptive sleep associations. He still wakes up occasionally at night, but settles back to sleep without parental intervention.

Chapter 4

Limit-Setting Disorder

WHEN A CHILD HAS a limit-setting disorder, she does not fall asleep at the desired time due to refusal to get ready for bed, stay in bed, or stay in the bedroom. She may have numerous demands for her parents for one more story, one more hug, one more drink of water. These demands, called curtain calls, are a way of stalling and avoiding getting ready for bed and going to sleep.

The result may be that your child gets her way — you stay with her until she falls asleep. Eventually, you may give in to her demands and stop setting a specific, consistent bedtime, allowing your child to fall asleep whenever and wherever she wants.

What Is Limit-Setting Disorder?

A limit-setting disorder occurs primarily in childhood when your child stalls or refuses to go to bed at a time you think is appropriate, with the result that you are not able to enforce a bedtime.

By about 9 months of age, a child understands the concept of object permanence. Until this age, a child does not understand that when parents are not seen (after falling asleep), they still exist. When a child develops this concept, she does not want the parent to be separated from her. That is the reason that you see stranger anxiety develop in children at this age.

Many children who have difficulty with settling at bedtime will also have difficulty with night wakings and do not sleep through the night. This exacerbates the problem at bedtime because the parents are chronically fatigued from the struggles at bedtime and from being woken frequently by their child through the night. For the child, the result may be inadequate sleep with increased irritability, decreased attention span, decreased school performance, and increased family tension.

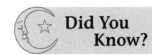

Did You Know?

Incidence
Limit-setting disorder is a common problem from 2 to 6 years of age. In several studies of healthy typically developing children, this difficulty with bedtime struggles is reported by parents consistently in about 5% to 10% of children.

WHAT THE TEXTBOOKS SAY

A limit-setting disorder is characterized by the following features:

- Your child does not want to go to sleep when you want him to. You or your partner recognizes this as a problem; however, your child may not.

- Setting limits becomes problematic when your child can climb out of his crib and is sleeping in a bed.

- Limits may be set, but only inconsistently and in an unpredictable manner.

- You may not know how to or do not recognize the importance of setting limits.

- This concern is usually limited to a young child. Your concern about setting limits at bedtime usually resolves when your child is old enough (typically in adolescence) to decide on his own bedtime, is aware of and responsible for the consequences of getting enough sleep, and lets you sleep.

(Based on the International Classification of Sleep Disorders, 2001)

Causes of Limit-Setting Disorder

There are parental and child factors that may contribute to a limit-setting disorder in children.

Parental Factors

- Parents lack the understanding of the importance of consistency in bedtime and wake time for children.

- Parents lack the knowledge of how to set limits, either being unable or unwilling to do this.

- Parents are inconsistent in setting limits both for sleep and for other activities.

- Parents feel guilty (parents who work long daytime hours can feel guilty about not spending enough time with their child and, therefore, do not enforce appropriate bedtimes, allowing more time together in the evening).

- Parents prioritize socializing with their child, rather than paying attention to the needs of the child at bedtime.

- Parents seek to avoid conflict with their child due to fatigue or other reasons.

- Parents are unable to agree on appropriate limits and do not set them as a result.

- Parents have their own emotional, psychiatric, or physical illness that interferes with their ability to set limits.

Child Factors

- The child does not have the same desire as the parent to go to sleep at night. The child would rather stay with parents, watch television, or read books, for example.

- The child does not have the capacity to understand the consequences on her behavior the next day if she does not get adequate sleep.

- The child wants additional parental attention, either because she does not get enough during the day or prefers the negative attention from an upset parent at night (when she makes demands) to no attention at all.

- The child has difficulty separating from parents.

- The child is put in bed too early because there is a mismatch between parents' desire for the child to go to sleep and child's ability to fall asleep at that time. This is common when the

---

case study: **Dorothy**

Mr. and Mrs. Campbell brought their daughter Dorothy to our sleep clinic because they could not get her to go to sleep easily. They have four children. The first three children did not cause any problems at bedtime. However, the fourth child, Dorothy, has been more challenging since the day she was born.

Dorothy was born prematurely at $7\frac{1}{2}$ months, weighing 1.8 kilograms (almost 4 pounds). She had to stay in the hospital for 4 weeks to gain weight. When she came home, her parents had to wake her every 2 to 3 hours for the first month at home to feed her. Her development was followed by a public health nurse and her doctor every 2 weeks to check on her weight gain until the age of 6 months.

Now, Dorothy is 4 years old. She is tiny and beautiful. She is treated by everyone in the family – parents, siblings, and grandmother (who lives in the family home) – like a little doll. She shares a room with her 6-year-old sister and at night, she will not go to sleep easily. At bedtime, Dorothy rules the family. She always demands from her tired parents one more drink, one more story, one more hug…and this can go on for an hour or more until she finally falls asleep. Once asleep, Dorothy sleeps through the night. During the day, she is also demanding of her parents, but she is easier to handle because they are not as tired. Nevertheless, Dorothy's parents recognized this was not a healthy sleep habit for her, with considerable effect on the health and happiness of the entire family….

(continued on page 131)

parents prefer a lark schedule (early to bed and early to rise) and the child prefers an owl schedule (later to bed and later to rise). The child may stay in bed and become more anxious about not falling asleep or, more commonly, cause problems by seeking attention.

- The child has incorrect sleep associations and has difficulty settling in bed because he hasn't learned to stay in bed alone and awake until he falls asleep.

- The child is taking medications that interfere with sleep onset.

- The child is anxious and has problems with separation in many settings, not just at bedtime. Further consultation with your health-care provider is needed to determine if the sleep problem can be resolved using the methods described in this book, if your child has an anxiety disorder, and if further counseling and evaluation are first required.

- The child may have a medical illness that causes more symptoms at night, such as nocturnal (nighttime) asthma and eczematous skin, which becomes itchier at night. These problems need to be addressed before trying to resolve the sleep problem.

- The child is experiencing recent stress or disruption, such as moving to a new home, separation of parents, or death in the family. These are not strictly behavioral causes and require further evaluation and consultation.

Guidelines for Treating Limit-Setting Disorder

PARENTS NEED TO SET limits and goals for their children around sleeping just as they do for other healthy habits, such as nutrition. You would not allow a 3-year-old child to choose what to eat without your direction. These are decisions that you make for your child. The same rule of thumb applies to sleep.

Children under the age of 6 to 7 need close adult supervision and guidance around sleep. Parents need to decide when, how, and where sleep takes place. Because these sleep decisions are made at a time when both the child and the parents are tired, parents may be tempted to defer to their child's wishes. When you are tired, it seems easier to avoid conflict by allowing your daughter to make choices about sleep that should be made by you as the parent.

STEP 1: Identify the Cause of the Disorder

If there are psychological or medical problems or recent acute stresses, discuss these issues with your health-care provider before attempting to resolve the problem on your own. If not, review the parent and child factors that may cause a limit-setting disorder and isolate the ones that apply to your behavior as a parent or your child's behavior.

STEP 2: Establish a Bedtime Routine

Establish and maintain a predictable, consistent bedtime each night. For establishing a bedtime routine, see Part 1, Chapter 3, "Sleep Hygiene."

STEP 3: Correct Sleep Associations

If your child has problems falling asleep and staying asleep related to incorrect sleep-onset associations, you need to deal with both these problems together. Learning to set limits will be part of the strategy you will need to teach your child better sleep habits and how to fall asleep alone. For strategies to treat incorrect sleep associations, see Part 3, Chapter 3, "Sleep-Onset Association Disorder."

STEP 4: Decrease Parental Attention

Aim to decrease the attention, positive and negative, to your child's demanding behavior at bedtime and during the night, if applicable. Talk to your health-care provider about how to set limits and reinforce them. They might recommend some of the following strategies:

Setting Limits, Rewards, and Consequences

1. Decide on reasonable limits. Children do well with structure and limits, and they will feel less anxious when they know what is expected.
2. Be consistent with the limits. Be consistent between parents and have other caregivers use the same limits consistently, if possible.
3. If your child is old enough to understand, talk to her during the day (not at bedtime when you are both tired) about what the changes/limits are. It will be helpful if your child knows in advance what the limits on her behavior are.
4. Do not try to make too many rules at once. Pick one challenge to work on at a time.
5. Make sure your child is looking at you and you have her attention when you tell him the rule/change/limit.

(6) Clearly state the rule or limit.

(7) Use positive reinforcement for good behavior. Praise her when she cooperates. Use a sticker chart or reward system to encourage cooperation.

(8) Decide ahead of time (with your child if she is old enough to understand) what the consequence will be for not cooperating.

STEP 5: Correct Sleep Phase Preferences

If your child is sleeping and waking too late or early with respect to a normal sleep schedule, this can be corrected after you have established limits at bedtime. You should put your child to bed when he is tired, even if this is later or earlier than desired. Once he is able to fall asleep in less than 30 minutes consistently, you can slowly adjust his schedule using the strategies described in the following chapter, Part 3, Chapter 5, "Circadian Rhythm Sleep Disorders."

Q. I believe that limits are important and when I'm home at night there is a set bedtime routine and bedtime. However when my partner is home and I'm out, the children stay up late and fall asleep when they are ready. My partner does not seem to understand the benefit of a proper bedtime. What should I do?

A. It is very important to have consistency between partners and other caregivers. Especially when you are establishing new routines, the more consistency there is, the easier it will be for your child. Sometimes, there will be unavoidable inconsistencies between adults, and your child will learn to adapt if your partner or other caregiver is at least consistent in their limits and expectations and you are consistent with yours.

Q. My child gets more angry and upset when I set limits at bedtime. It's just easier for me to let him sleep in my bed than to have him upset himself and the whole family. How do I set limits without making him more upset?

A. Although your child will be more upset when you initially establish limits, he will actually benefit from the structure and knowing the expectations regarding his behavior. It may be easier to give in to his demands and let him go to sleep in your bed, but if you (or your partner) are unhappy with this arrangement, then it is important to try and change it. If you are having trouble with setting limits, you should talk to your health-care provider to determine how to resolve the problem.

case study: **Dorothy** (continued)

Dorothy's parents were able to identify that they felt more protective toward her because of her premature start to life. Once they could recognize this, they were able to change their pattern of giving in to her demands at night.

First, they established a bedtime routine. This became a special time for Dorothy, away from her three siblings. She was alone in her room with either her mother or father. During the routine, Dorothy's mother or father read her a story and at the end of the story, the parent reinforces that it will be time for bed. Dorothy is allowed to make one request only, for a drink, another short story, or a hug, and then parents leave her in her room to fall asleep.

If Dorothy cooperates, she receives a sticker, and when she has five stickers, she has a special outing to the park to play. If she doesn't cooperate, her parents use the door-closing routine to keep her in her room, intermittently checking on her until she falls asleep.

After a few weeks, Dorothy no longer needed these reinforcements because she learned what the limits were at bedtime and went to sleep more easily. She is not perfect (which would not be expected) and still has nights when she is more demanding than her parents would like. However, her parents learned to set limits, and if needed, they can go back to a routine with positive reinforcement and consequences if she does not cooperate at bedtime.

Chapter 5

Circadian Rhythm Sleep Disorders (Delayed and Advanced Sleep Phase Syndrome)

WHAT HAPPENS IF OWLS and larks try to live together in one family? If you are a lark (with a preference for an early to bed and early to rise schedule) and your child is an owl (with a preference for a late to bed and late to rise schedule), how can you manage to coexist happily in the same household? Some children have an early or late preference, but manage to get enough sleep and wake up in the morning easily. However, some children (and adults) have difficulty obtaining adequate sleep due to their delayed or advanced sleep phase preference. When they are unable to function, missing school or work because of this preference, it is called a circadian rhythm sleep disorder. The most common type is the delayed sleep phase syndrome.

Did You Know?

Sleep Maintenance
We have two processes that maintain our sleep and wake cycles — the homeostatic drive, which is like a sleep pressure that builds up the longer we are awake, and the circadian rhythm, which regulates the timing of sleep and wake. When our circadian rhythm is disrupted, it can lead to a delay or advance in our sleep cycle.

What Is a Circadian Rhythm Sleep Disorder?

A circadian rhythm disorder is when you have normal sleep quantity and quality, but you are sleeping and waking at the 'wrong' time. Your body is not synchronized with the normal patterns of body temperature, melatonin, and other hormones released in a predictable pattern every 24 hours.

WHAT THE TEXTBOOKS SAY

Several circadian rhythms occur in the body based on a daily cycle of about every 24 hours:

- Our sleep-wake cycle (we sleep and wake every 24 hours)

- Our core body temperature (which rises and falls predictably every 24 hours, with the lowest time in our temperature being around 3:00 to 4:30 in the morning)

- Release in the brain of the hormone melatonin (triggered by darkness each night and one of the factors that aids in sleep induction)

- Release of other hormones, such as growth hormone and cortisol (in a cyclical way each 24 hours)

If your child prefers a much later or earlier bedtime and wake time than customary, and this interferes with daytime functioning, causing excessive daytime sleepiness, your child has a sleep disorder. A delay of 3 to 6 hours in your preferred bedtime and wake time is called a delayed sleep phase syndrome; an advance of the same time is called an advanced sleep phase syndrome.

Biological Clock

Each day, we adjust our biological clock so that our bodies and rhythms do not drift out of phase with a 24-hour day by using cues from the environment. The strongest cue to our clock is light. Sunlight, especially in the morning, acts like an alarm to our internal clock. Taking away light at night (or being in a dark environment) is the cue that it is time to go to sleep.

If you are exposed to light at the right time (in the morning), this helps to set your clock properly, and if you are exposed to light at the wrong time (in the evening) this disrupts your clock. Take, for example, a teenager who falls asleep at a very late time, around 2:00 or 3:00 a.m., and then sleeps in a darkened room until noon. He misses being exposed to morning light, and if he misses this cue for many days, he may develop a delayed sleep phase syndrome, each day only being able to fall asleep late and preferring to wake up late. If he is able to wake up on time for school, this is with great difficulty, and he is excessively sleepy from getting inadequate hours of sleep. The delayed sleep phase syndrome is the most common circadian rhythm disorder, and along with the advanced sleep phase syndrome, can cause sleep problems in children and adolescents.

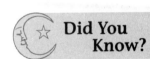

Did You Know?

Light Sensitivity
Light is an important clue to set the biologic clock. People who are blind, wear dark sunglasses at all times, do not have exposure to natural outdoor light, or live in some geographic areas where the light-dark cycle is altered, such as the polar regions of the Earth, may experience an altered sleep phase.

TYPES OF CIRCADIAN RHYTHM SLEEP DISORDERS

There are six types of circadian rhythm disorders, but the most common in children and teenagers is delayed sleep phase syndrome and, less common, advanced sleep phase syndrome.

1. Delayed sleep phase syndrome

2. Advanced sleep phase syndrome

3. Non-24-hour sleep-wake syndrome

4. Irregular or disorganized sleep-wake pattern

5. Change in rhythm caused by working shifts

6. Change in rhythm caused by jet lag

Normal, Advanced, and Delayed Sleep Phases

Sleep Phase Preferences

In itself, being a morning person or evening person is not a problem. Your child can be either a night owl or a morning lark without having a sleep disorder. The key is obtaining adequate sleep at night and functioning well during the day. Being a night owl or a morning lark becomes a problem when this preference affects your child's ability to cope with his own daily life and the lives of his family members, including his parents.

Adolescent Preference

Teenagers tend to be become night owls for several reasons. Their biological clock seems to prefer a later bedtime. If your teenager has a period of time when he is studying late at night, socializing, or working late shifts, he may develop a sleep phase delay pattern. Using the computer, watching television, playing video games, using the Internet, or talking on the phone may contribute to adolescents delaying bedtime and developing a delayed sleep phase preference. During vacations, teenagers may develop this preference when there are no time constraints or need to sleep and wake at the expected times. Teenagers often delay their meals, eating late in the morning and late in the evening, which reinforces their sleep delay. Eating or drinking foods or beverages with caffeine, drinking alcohol, and using illegal drugs may also contribute to sleep delay in adolescents.

Did You Know?

Alert in the Morning
If your child feels most alert in the morning, but has difficulty going to sleep, he may have sleep-onset insomnia, but probably does not have a delayed sleep phase syndrome. Children with a delayed sleep phase feel less alert in the morning and more alert later in the day.

Advanced, Normal, and Delayed Sleep Phases

This graph illustrates normal, advanced, and delayed sleep phases for a typical 10 hours of sleep a night. If you sleep according to any of these phases, you should be able to function, although the person who sleeps at the normal time may feel the most rested. In most cases of a delayed or advanced sleep phase, the person does not sleep for an adequate time. For example, the teenager who falls asleep after midnight, then wakens at 6:00 or 7:00 a.m. for school, does not get adequate sleep.

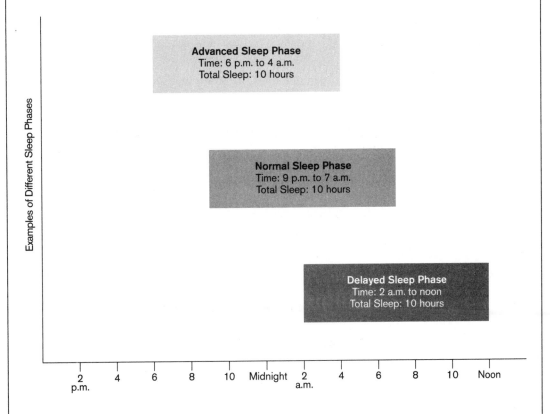

Symptoms of Advanced Sleep Phase

- Misses evening activities

- Can't stay awake after dinner and wakes too early

- Meal schedule advanced earlier than desired

Symptoms of Delayed Sleep Phase

- Unable to fall asleep at desired bedtime or to wake in morning

- Misses exposure to sunlight in the morning

- Meal schedule delayed and breakfast often skipped

MORNINGNESS/EVENINGNESS QUESTIONNAIRE

This questionnaire was used in a research study of children in Grades 4 to 6 by Dr. Mary Carskadon and her colleagues to determine if more physically mature students (those in later stages of puberty) were more likely to have a morning or an evening sleep phase preference. You can use this scale with your child and ask him to complete the questions to see if he prefers the morning (more of a lark type) or the evening (more of an owl type). Most children, though not all, will show a preference for the evening pattern as they go through puberty. An adolescent who is more advanced in the physical changes associated with puberty may have a stronger evening (or owl type) preference than one who is not yet as advanced.

Instructions

Ask your child to answer the questions by circling the answer she feels best describes her preference.

1. Imagine: School is canceled! You can get up whenever you want to. When would you get out of bed? Between...

a. 5:00 and 6:30 a.m.

b. 6:30 and 7:45 a.m.

c. 7:45 and 9:45 a.m.

d. 9:45 and 11:00 a.m.

e. 11:00 a.m. and noon

2. Is it easy for you to get up in the morning?

a. No way!

b. Sort of

c. Pretty easy

d. It's a cinch

3. Gym class is set for 7:00 in the morning. How do you think you'll do?

a. My best!

b. Okay

c. Worse then usual

d. Awful

4. The bad news: you have to take a two-hour test. The good news: you can take it when you think you'll do your best. What time it that?

a. 8:00 to 10:00 a.m.

b. 1:00 a.m. to 1:00 p.m.

c. 3:00 to 5:00 p.m.

d. 7:00 to 9:00 p.m.

5. When do you have the most energy to do your favorite things?

a. Morning! I'm tired in the evening

b. Morning more then evening

c. Evening more then morning

d. Evening! I'm tired in the morning

6. Guess what? Your parents have decided to let you set your own bedtime. What time would you pick? Between...

a. 8:00 and 9:00 p.m.

b. 9:00 and 10:15 p.m.

c. 10:15 p.m. and 12:30 a.m.

d. 12:30 and 1:45 a.m.

e. 1:45 and 3:00 a.m.

7. How alert are you in the first half hour that you're up?

a. Out of it

b. A little dazed

c. Okay

d. Ready to take on the world

8. When does your body start to tell you it's time for bed (even if you ignore it)? Between...

a. 8:00 and 9:00 p.m.

b. 9:00 and 10:15 p.m.

c. 10:15 p.m. and 12:30 a.m.

d. 12:30 and 1:45 a.m.

e. 1:45 and 3:00 a.m.

9. Say you had to get up at 6:00 a.m. every morning: What would you be like?

a. Awful

b. Not so great

c. Okay (if I have to)

d. Fine, no problem

10. When you wake up in the morning, how long does it take for you to be totally "with it?"

a. 0 to 10 minutes

b. 11 to 20 minutes

c. 21 to 40 minutes

d. More then 40 minutes

Scoring

To determine your child's morning or evening preference, give points to the questions as follows:

Questions 2, 7, 9: a-1, b-2, c-3, d-4, e-5

Questions 1, 3, 4, 5, 6, 8, 10: a-5, b-4, c-3, d-2, e-1

If your child's score is high (with 42 being the highest), then he is more of a lark type (who prefers an early bedtime and early wake time).

If your child's score is low (with 14 being the lowest) then he is more of an owl type (who prefers a late bedtime and a late wake time).

If your child falls in the middle, he is not strongly preferring the morning or evening. This does not necessarily mean that your child has a sleep phase syndrome – only a sleep phase preference.

What Is Delayed Sleep Phase Syndrome?

In delayed sleep phase syndrome, the major sleep episode is delayed in relation to the desired clock time, resulting in symptoms of sleep-onset insomnia or difficulty in awakening at the desired time. Delayed sleep phase syndrome can be seen at any age, but usually starts in adolescence and may affect 5% to 10% of teenagers.

Symptoms of Delayed Sleep Phase Syndrome
Checklist 1

Check for these symptoms to determine if your child has a delayed sleep phase syndrome, a true sleep disorder, and is not simply an owl type with a delayed sleep phase preference.

❑ Your child prefers to go to bed 3 to 6 hours later than you want.

❑ When your child goes to bed at his preferred time, he is able to fall asleep easily.

❑ When your child goes to bed at your expected time, he is unable to fall asleep.

❑ Once asleep, your child sleeps well and does not wake at night.

❑ Your child prefers to wake 3 to 6 hours later than he needs to.

❑ When you are able to wake your child up at your desired time, he is very sleepy, especially in the morning but can be sleepy throughout the day.

WHAT THE TEXTBOOKS SAY

Delayed sleep phase syndrome is characterized by the following features:

- Your child falls asleep and wakens consistently later than desired.

- Although these times are later than desired, it is nearly the same time every day

- Once your child is asleep, he has little or no difficulty staying asleep.

- Your child has a lot of trouble waking at a desired (normal) time in the morning.

- Even if you consistently try to have your child in bed and waking at desired times, he is unable to advance his sleep phase to a normal schedule.

(Based on the International Classification of Sleep Disorders, 2001)

CONSEQUENCES OF DELAYED SLEEP PHASE SYNDROME

Bedtime struggles: Your child will not be able to fall asleep at the expected time.

Morning struggles: Your child will not be able to wake up at the expected time in the morning.

Weekend catch up: If your child has a true delayed sleep phase syndrome, he will not be able to just sleep late and catch up on his sleep debt on the weekend. This will just enforce his inability to fall asleep on Sunday night and lead to the same problems on Monday morning of not being able to wake up.

Inadequate sleep: if your child has this syndrome but you are able to get him out of bed to attend school, he will be tired due to the lack of sleep.

- ❐ Your child seems to be the most awake in the late afternoon to early morning hours.
- ❐ Your child often does not eat his first meal until 3 to 6 hours after breakfast time.
- ❐ Your child prefers eating late at night.
- ❐ On the weekends, if allowed, your child will wake at his preferred time, after 12 p.m.
- ❐ On holidays, when he is allowed to sleep and wake on his own schedule, your child keeps a fairly regular, but later than desired schedule and is well rested.
- ❐ Your child may lack motivation to change this delayed sleep pattern. This will need to be discussed either at home or with your health-care provider because you will not be able to help your teenager change this pattern without him being motivated to do so.

Checklist 2

Check off these symptoms to determine if your child has other problems that may contribute to delayed sleep phase preference, delayed sleep phase syndrome, or another sleep disorder.

- ❐ Your child eats foods or drinks beverages with caffeine, smokes cigarettes, or uses street drugs. Adolescents may use these substances for many reasons, but they will likely interfere with wake and sleeping rhythms and may promote delayed sleep phase syndrome.

❐ Your child is experiencing a mood or psychiatric disorder. The symptoms of a delayed sleep phase may be part of a mental health disorder, diagnosed or undiagnosed.

❐ Your child is experiencing social problems or school refusal. Your teenager may develop this syndrome as a way to avoid a problematic social, work, or school environment.

What Is Advanced Sleep Phase Syndrome?

If your child has an advanced phase syndrome, his preferred bedtime and wake time will be 3 to 6 hours earlier than desired. Once asleep, he will be able to sleep through the night. This is a much less common problem than delayed sleep phase syndrome, especially in adolescents because of the biologic changes that promote a later bedtime.

Symptoms of Advanced Sleep Phase Syndrome

If you recognize the following symptoms of advanced sleep phase syndrome in your child and it is a new pattern that has recently developed, you should discuss this with your health-care

case history: Rachel

Rachel, a 16-year-old student, came to our clinic complaining that she was tired most days. She was not able to fall asleep until 3:00 a.m. most nights, even though she was in her room by midnight. She would start her homework typically at 10:30 p.m. From 10:30 to 3 a.m., she would do her homework, play on the computer, listen to music, and chat on the Internet. She had found a whole group of friends electronically who had the same schedule, so there was always someone to talk to on the Internet in the early morning hours. Finally, she would fall asleep at 3:00 a.m. and then have great difficulty waking at 7:00 a.m. for school.

As a result, she often missed school, but because she was a good student, she managed to achieve good grades by following the homework of her peers. On the weekends, Rachel liked to stay out late with friends, getting to sleep around 3:00 a.m. and waking at noon. She felt somewhat less tired on the weekends, but still was not happy with her schedule because she never really felt awake and alert all day...

(continued on page 148)

provider to ensure there are no medical problems or other disorders present before attempting to change your child's sleep behavior.

❐ Your child can't stay awake until bedtime.

❐ Your child can't stay asleep to an expected morning time, but wakes in the early morning.

❐ Your child's sleep is of normal quality and quantity, but earlier than desired.

❐ Your child wakens spontaneously in the morning.

❐ Your child is most alert in the morning.

❐ Your child is able to get enough sleep if he stays on his schedule and will not be excessively sleepy during the day.

❐ Your child is unable to participate in any activities in the early evening due to his need for an early bedtime.

Guidelines for Treating Delayed Sleep Phase Syndrome

IF THE FOLLOWING BEHAVIOR-BASED guidelines for treating delayed sleep phase syndrome do not work, you should discuss this problem with your health-care provider. Sometimes other therapies, such as taking melatonin, using artificial bright light, or chronotherapy (making gradual adjustments to the sleep phase by delaying sleep) may help. The use of melatonin at night and bright-light therapy in the morning for treating adults has been studied, but further research with children and adolescents is needed before these treatments can be recommended. Discuss these therapies with your health-care provider, who may refer you to a sleep specialist. There may also be an underlying problem with substance abuse, school avoidance, depression, or other social and emotional difficulties. Referral to someone in the area of mental health may be needed.

Care of Younger Children

In a younger child who prefers a later-than-desired bedtime, you need to first identify if, in addition to a phase delay, she also has other problems resulting in sleeplessness, such as sleep-onset association disorder or limit-setting disorder. The first issues to address are these, while allowing her to fall asleep at her preferred bedtime, even if it is later than desired. Once the other problems are improving and your child is able to fall asleep alone and sleep through the night, then you can gradually move her bedtime and wake time earlier until she is able to sleep and wake at a desired time.

Care of Adolescents

It is common for teenagers to develop a delayed sleep preference because they are biologically predisposed to this as puberty advances naturally. When extreme, this evening preference can interfere with school attendance. Alternatively, your teenager may wake up for school but have daytime fatigue from inadequate sleep. You can help your child resolve this problem if she is motivated. However, if there are other issues contributing to her phase delay, such as depression, school avoidance or substance abuse, your health-care provider should further evaluate and help you to manage these problems.

STEP 1: Determine the Causes

If your child is not a teenager, it is likely that he has developed the delayed sleep phase syndrome as a result of another behavior-based problem, such as limit-setting disorder or sleep-onset association disorder. The biological change that precipitates this syndrome begins in early adolescence, so there is unlikely to be a biological basis to a young child developing a sleep phase problem. If the problem is a true delayed sleep phase, follow the routine outlined here for a teenager.

STEP 2: Educate Your Child and Family

If your teenager has a delayed sleep phase syndrome, the most important treatment is educating your teenager and your family about the symptoms, causes, and consequences of this disorder. Encourage your child to read this chapter and to complete the morningness/eveningness questionnaire. If your teenager understands the problem and can be motivated to change his behavior, it will be easier to resolve.

STEP 3: Motivate Your Child to Change

Discuss the following motivational strategies with your child, which may help his decision to change his sleep phase preference. Consider using appropriate rewards and consequences. These strategies and rewards should be agreed upon by you and your child. Consider documenting these discussions in writing and referring to the document later as needed.

1. Set limits about expected behavior regarding evening activities, curfews, bedtimes, school attendance and performance, and changes to improve sleep behavior.

2. Develop a system of positive reinforcement for complying with the proposed changes. This may include such activities as time on the computer and social outings. They will need to be tailored to your child's interests and age.

3. Make agreements between you and your child about consequences for failure to comply with changes. For the older adolescent who wants to obtain or has a driver's license, it is appropriate to establish this as a

reward (for example, driving lessons or the use of the car) or consequence (loss of these privileges) for improved sleep behavior. Drowsy driving, at all ages, but especially in a young inexperienced driver, is a dangerous situation.

4. Establish a system so that you can ensure that your child is complying with the sleep-wake changes. For example, if you leave for work in the morning before your teenager gets up for school, develop a system to ensure that he wakens on time and gets to school. He can call you when he wakens and again when he is on his way to school. Another alternative, if more adult supervision is needed, would be to meet with the school office personnel and for a predetermined period of time, ask someone in the school office to check each morning that he arrives at school on time.

STEP 4: Improve Sleep Hygiene

Make sure your child has good sleep hygiene. Ensure that she has a good sleep environment. This means a safe, comfortable room without a computer, television, or telephone (or with these turned off at bedtime). The bedroom should be comfortable, cool, and quiet at night, with little or no artificial light. Review Part 1, Chapter 3, "Sleep Hygiene," and pay attention especially to some habits that contribute to a delayed sleep phase syndrome: lack of sunlight in the morning, lack of regular breakfasts and late evening meals, and use of caffeine and other substances that act as stimulants and contribute to sleep-onset insomnia.

STEP 5: Establish a Relaxing Bedtime Routine

Develop a routine with your teenager's input. Don't try to impose or enforce your preferred routine without explaining it to your child. Get him to 'buy in'.

STEP 6: Keep a Sleep Diary

Help your child to keep a sleep diary for 2 weeks so that you can estimate his average sleep and wake times. See Part 2, Chapter 3, "Treatment of Sleep Disorders," for guidelines on keeping a sleep diary.

STEP 7: Reset Your Child's Biological Clock

The following suggestions are for teenagers who are sleeping late in the morning and missing school or work. By resetting your child's biological clock, you can slowly move his sleeping schedule earlier until he is able to fall asleep and wake at a desired time. This can be done by noting what time your teenager wakes in the morning, and then slightly depriving your teenager of sleep by moving the wake time earlier without changing his actual bedtime. Your child can go to sleep when he is sleepy, even if it is not the desired bedtime. Don't worry about the bedtime initially.

1. To start, decide with your teenager an appropriate time to wake up in the morning. This should be about 30 minutes earlier than his usual wake time. Temporarily, this may have to be later than desired, but it should be a regular time every morning, 7 days a week.

2. Let your teenager take responsibility for setting his alarm and waking up at an earlier time for 1 week. If he tries to do this, and can't wake up on his own, then decide ahead of time how you will help him wake up. Because the wake time will be earlier than his usual or desired time, he will be mildly sleep deprived after 1 week.

3. At the end of the week, move his bedtime back by 30 minutes. Have your teenager start the bedtime routine 30 minutes before the desired bedtime. For this week, he will get into bed 30 minutes earlier, and continue with the same rise time, 30 minutes earlier than his baseline waking time.

4. Now, alternate moving the waking time earlier by another 30 minutes for 1 week, then the bedtime earlier by 30 minutes for 1 week until he is at the desired bedtime and wake time.

5. While making these changes, the most important step to enforce is the waking time. You can ensure that your teenager develops a good bedtime routine and tries to get to sleep at the correct time, but you cannot make someone actually fall asleep. As long as he continues to wake at the time you have agreed upon and does not nap during the day, he will begin to be able to fall asleep at an earlier bedtime also.

6. Pay attention to morning and evening light and meals. When your teenager wakes up in the morning, encourage him to get exposure to sunlight and to eat breakfast. In the evening, he should be in dim light for several hours before bedtime and avoid heavy meals late at night. This will also help reinforce the changes in his schedule.

7. Once he has achieved the desired sleep and wake time, your child must continue with this schedule for 6 weeks to reset his biological clock. He needs to know before starting this routine that he will not have more energy and less fatigue during the day immediately after changing his routine. It will take about 6 weeks before he will notice a difference.

8. It will be hard for your teenager to keep this schedule, especially getting into bed and waking earlier than he is used to on the weekends. After 6 weeks on this schedule, your child can relax the schedule 1 night a week (for example, on the weekend) to participate in late-night social, work, or recreational activities.

9. Make sure that your teenager understands before starting this change in routine that eventually (after the first 6 weeks), when he has developed a new schedule and no longer has a phase delay problem,

he can resume normal teenage habits, socializing with his friends late on weekend nights.

10. Once your child has experienced a significant sleep phase delay problem, he may be prone to lapses from his new, normal sleep-wake schedule, especially on the weekend. To avoid this from happening, encourage him to wake up on Sunday morning earlier than desired to ensure that he can get to sleep on Sunday night, ready for school or work challenges on Monday.

Resetting the Biological Clock

This sketch provides a step-by-step guide on how to move the waking time earlier, which slightly shortens the actual sleep time, causing mild sleep deprivation, then how to move the bedtime back. Your child will be able to fall asleep earlier because he will be a bit sleep deprived.

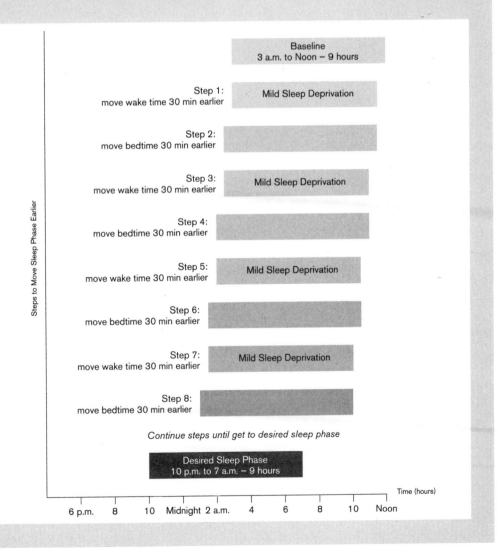

Tips for Resetting Your Child's Biological Clock

1. Expose your child to sunlight in the morning and provide a dark room for sleeping: If you have the option in your home, you may even want to move him to another bedroom in your home with good early morning sun exposure.

2. Make sure your child understands that he will not feel better in 2 or 3 days: It will take about 6 weeks before he will actually feel more alert during the day. You can explain that this pattern took months or years to develop and will take some time to adjust. In fact, he may actually feel more tired temporarily as he is trying to shorten his sleep by waking up early so that he will be sleep deprived and be able to move his sleep-onset time backward.

3. Let your child get into bed when he is tired: If he is unable to fall asleep after about 20 minutes, he should get out of bed, do a quiet activity, and then after 20 minutes get back into bed and try to fall asleep. See Part 3, Chapter 15, "Teenage Sleepiness," for other tips on treating sleep-onset insomnia in teenagers.

4. Use the bedroom only for sleeping: Don't allow your teenager to use the bedroom for anything except sleeping, including watching television, listening to music, or using the computer. This rule can be relaxed in the future when the sleep problem resolves.

5. No naps during the day: If your child has a daytime nap while trying to adjust his sleep phase, he will have more difficulty getting to sleep (sleep-onset insomnia). He is waking up somewhat earlier to cause slight sleep deprivation so he will be more tired during the day. However, a nap will only make it harder for him to comply with the changing routine. If he naps while trying to change the schedule, it will be easier and more likely that he will stay up late at night, thus reinforcing the delayed sleep schedule.

6. Stay on schedule: Once your teenager has adjusted to the schedule, he needs to stay on it for the next 6 weeks. However, he can wake 1 hour later on the weekend days than on the weekdays.

7. Exercise: Exercise is very helpful to promote sleep onset and deeper sleep. Some people find that exercising late in the day contributes to sleep-onset insomnia. If this is the case for your child, then he should exercise in the morning or early afternoon, rather than in the late afternoon or evening.

Guidelines for Treating Advanced Sleep Phase Syndrome

To TREAT A CHILD with an advanced phase, the treatment is similar to the delayed phase, but in reverse.

STEP 1: Improve Sleep Hygiene

Review the tips on sleep hygiene in Part 1, Chapter 3, "Sleep Hygiene." Establish a bedtime routine and a scheduled bedtime.

STEP 2: Encourage Change in the Morning

You cannot force your child to sleep later if he has an advanced phase and a preference for an early waking time. However, you can consider the reinforcement activities that occur in the early morning that may encourage him to develop this habit. For example, if your child crawls into bed with you and turns on the television, or you get up with him to play, read stories or give him breakfast, all these activities are helping to continue his preference for early morning awaking. In order to help him move his wake time until later, limit the positive interaction and delay breakfast.

STEP 3: Encourage Change in the Evening

You will be able to gradually move the bedtime later if you do this in small increments. After moving the bedtime later slowly and decreasing the positive interactions in the morning hours, you can slowly advance his schedule to a more desirable sleep and wake time.

STEP 4: Keep a Sleep Diary

Record your child's sleep-onset time and waking time in a sleep diary for 2 weeks so that you can estimate his average sleep and wake times. For guidelines on keeping a sleep diary, see Part 2, Chapter 2, "Treatment of Sleep Disorders."

STEP 5: Reset Your Child's Biological Clock

During a 2-week period, gradually delay bedtime by 15 to 30 minutes and increase the delay every 4 to 5 days. Delay breakfast and the time that your child can get out of bed by the same increments.

STEP 6: Set Limits and Offer Rewards

You cannot force your child to sleep, so you need to establish limits for what quiet activities he can do in his room (for example, reading a book, playing with a puzzle, but not waking you) until the time you have agreed upon. You can use a reward system to help your child stay in his room in the morning.

Q. What determines if my child has a simple phase preference (to be a lark or an owl) or a sleep disorder — a delayed or an advanced sleep phase syndrome?

A. There is a difference between the child who just prefers a later bedtime and wake time (or earlier), but functions well at school without any sign of excessive daytime sleepiness and the child who has a circadian rhythm sleep disorder. It is normal to be a bit of an owl or a lark. If, however, your child's preference for sleep time is so advanced or delayed that he is not getting enough sleep (in the case of the owl who has to get up for school) or missing activities in the evening (in the case of the lark who goes to bed after supper), then this is more of a disorder than a simple preference.

Q. We tend to be night owls but our child is a morning lark. How do we manage this?

A. You may think that your child has a sleep problem if he doesn't match with your sleep preference, but if you were larks, this would not be a problem. Because some of the tendency toward being an evening or morning person is hereditary, he may have inherited this tendency from his grandparents. You may not be able to change your child's sleep phase preference and will need to adapt to his different biologic needs to ensure he is getting adequate sleep and functions well during the day. Likewise, parents will need to adapt to the sleep preference of a night owl child if they are morning larks.

case study: **Rachel** (continued)

Rachel was motivated to change her schedule when she recognized she was not functioning well at home or at school. She also wanted to learn to drive.

We recommended that Rachel keep a sleep diary for 2 weeks. It looked as though her bedtime was consistently 3:00 a.m. and her preferred waking time was noon, which resulted in 9 hours of sleep. We then set up a schedule to realign her sleeping with a more normal pattern.

Rachel and her parents agreed that if she could wake and sleep at a more desirable schedule, her reward would be driving lessons.

After the first 6 weeks of moving her waking time and then her bedtime alternatively earlier, she managed to keep a fairly regular schedule. She is now learning how to drive.

Chapter 6

Excessive Crying

ALL BABIES CRY, which can disturb their sleep and yours when excessive. Crying is the best way they have to communicate with the world and with their parents in particular. Babies cry for all kinds of reasons — to let us know they are hungry, wet, lonely, tired, bored, frustrated…the list goes on. While you understand that your baby will cry a certain amount, you expect you will be able to help her stop crying when you feed her, change her diaper, or comfort her. Sometimes, there is nothing you can do to stop the crying. Excessive crying is unpredictable and seems to go on and on. This sense of helplessness in the face of excessive crying is perhaps the most troubling experience of being a parent. We all want our babies to be settled and content.

What Causes Excessive Crying?

Excessive crying is not always bad. This is your baby's way of telling you he is hungry, overly tired, or suffering an illness. Excessive crying may also be caused by colic or temperament. When your child and you experience chronic sleep disturbance or sleep deprivation, excessive crying becomes problematic.

Hunger

It is normal for your baby to cry if he is hungry; however, if he seems to be always crying from hunger and he is not gaining weight, then you may have a problem in how you are feeding him or he may have a significant medical problem.

Overtired

If your baby is not getting enough sleep and is overtired, his crying may increase. A young baby (until the age of 2 to 3 months) will generally fall asleep between 1½ and 2 hours after his feeding time. Most newborns need to sleep about 16 to 18 out of 24 hours and 14 to 16 hours at 2 months of age. Some babies will sleep less or more than the average. You should talk to your health-care provider about your baby's sleep need if he is crying excessively and sleeping less than average.

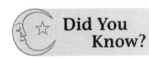

Did You Know?

Crying Studies
In surveys, 20% of parents report a problem with young infants crying or being irritable. Crying usually is at its worst at 6 weeks of age, but lessens or stops by 12 to 16 weeks of age. Crying can occur throughout the day, but tends to be worse in the evening.

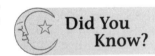

Did You Know?

Hunger Signs
Frequent, short feedings may be a sign of your baby being hungry. If you are concerned that your baby is crying due to hunger, consult with your health-care provider.

Medical Conditions

Sometimes, excessive crying is caused by common medical conditions, such as ear infections, heartburn (gastroesophageal reflux), or more serious conditions. Be sure to consult with your doctor if your child begins to cry excessively, especially if this is new behavior.

Colic and Temperament

About 95% of babies who are described by parents as crying excessively are healthy without any medical cause for their crying. If hunger, fatigue, and medical problems can be ruled out as the cause of excessive crying, your baby may be crying due to colic or a particular temperament that makes him a 'fussy baby'. Colic and temperament can be treated with behavior intervention, offering the frustrated parent and crying child much needed rest.

What Is Colic?

The medical definition of colic is a rule of three: the crying occurs for 3 hours or more a day, on 3 days or more a week, and for at least 3 weeks. The bouts of crying last for long periods of time, and are often clustered in the late afternoon or early evening, not just at sleep times.

Even if your baby isn't crying quite this much or hasn't been crying for quite that long, periods of lengthy crying are difficult and heartbreaking for even the most patient of parents. Every baby is unique, and there is a wide variation between babies in terms of how much each one cries. Babies in the same family can be very different; one baby may have cried very little in the early months, while his sister began crying for long periods of time very early on.

Parental Reaction

Colic is one of the toughest things a parent can deal with in the early months of a baby's life. Although you are working very hard to keep your baby settled, nothing seems to work, and you don't get the reward of a happy, smiling baby. To see and hear your baby so distressed may leave you feeling helpless, angry, and guilty. However, a baby with colic is not a reflection on you as a parent — your baby's crying is not your fault and it does not mean that you're a bad parent. Nor does it mean that there is something wrong with your baby. Excessive crying in the first few months is so common among babies that health-care professionals do not call this behavior abnormal.

Did You Know?

Heartburn?
Researchers have examined babies who look like they are having stomach or heartburn (reflux) problems because they have a red face, pull up their legs, or pass wind. It has been shown that these behaviors are more likely to be part of normal crying than related to stomach or heartburn problems.

Did You Know?

Colic Duration
Excessive crying from colic usually appears within the first few weeks of life, peaks at about 6 weeks of age, and gradually tapers off, disappearing usually by age 3 or 4 months.

SYMPTOMS OF COLIC

If your baby has colic, you may recognize the following symptoms. Check off any that you observe.

☐ Babies with colic often draw their legs up to their belly or alternate between pulling their legs up and stretching them out straight, may get red in the face, clench their fists and have a facial expression as though they are in pain.

☐ Some infants refuse to eat or appear to become fussy shortly after eating. A colicky baby seems to be distressed, not just frustrated, angry, or hungry.

☐ It is difficult to ease a colicky baby's distress by any simple intervention. If your baby settles simply by picking her up out of the crib or by rocking her, this is likely not colic.

Long-Term Consequences

It may help you to know that babies who have colic do not have any more problems with their development or intelligence than babies who cry very little. There do not seem to be any long-term effects of excessive crying. Nor does it mean that if your baby cries a lot in the first few months, this behavior will continue in the future. Babies do eventually outgrow their crying and go on to be healthy, happy babies. You may be relieved to know that many parents feel the same way and have the same challenges with their colicky baby.

Causes of Colic

No one really knows what causes colic, but there is no shortage of old wives' tales about colic. Some have speculated that colic is caused by acid reflux or heartburn; however, it is unlikely that your baby is crying because he suffers from gastroesophageal reflux unless he is crying and vomiting frequently.

Food allergies have also been proposed as a cause, but very few babies have a true food allergy, especially breast-fed babies. If your baby's excessive crying is also associated with swelling, itching, wheezing, a constantly stuffy nose, vomiting, or a rash, your health-care provider may suggest eliminating cow's milk from your diet if you are breast-feeding, or switching to a soy or hypoallergenic formula if you are bottle-feeding your baby.

It has been suggested that colic may be related to an immaturity of the nervous system, an immaturity of the digestive system, or simply a difficult infant temperament, but no single explanation seems to fit.

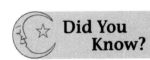

Did You Know?

Crying It Out
If your baby does have colic, a 'crying it out' approach is usually not effective with colicky babies and may increase the number of crying bouts and length of their crying. Studies show that crying episodes are shorter in babies who are carried more and breast-fed on demand.

case study: **Sonja**

Sonja is a healthy, 2-month-old baby girl, but her parents, Joe and Maria, came to our clinic complaining that they cannot get her to stop crying. She is a very special baby – Maria is 42 years old and Sonja is the product of years of fertility treatment.

When Sonja cries, only movement seems to console her. She will settle somewhat if she is rocked, walked, or taken for a car ride. She wakes up crying, and although she is at her loudest in the late afternoon and evening, she seems inconsolable 24 hours a day.

Her parents report that when she is crying, her face turns red, she pulls up her legs, and looks like she is distressed from pain. Sonja sleeps about 13 out of 24 hours. Joe and Maria are desperate to find a way to manage Sonja's apparently irritable temperament....

(continued on page 157)

Guidelines for Treating Colic

BECAUSE THE EXACT causes of colic remain a mystery, the treatment for colic is not straightforward. The strategies that work to reduce one baby's crying may not be effective for all parents.

STEP 1: Rule Out Common Causes

Rule out the usual reasons for crying, such as being hungry, overtired, or uncomfortable because of clothing. Also rule out medical conditions with the help of your doctor.

STEP 2: Keep a Crying Diary

Record each time your baby has a crying spell, noting when they occur and what activities or events are going on when the crying begins. You may be able to detect a pattern of what triggers bouts of crying. Knowing what sets your baby off can help you plan ahead to prevent or reduce crying spells before they get too bad.

STEP 3: Reduce Stimulation

Minimize stimulation around your baby. Bright lights, noise, or a large number of people may overstimulate your baby and aggravate the crying. Try to recognize early warning signs that crying is beginning and reduce stimulation right away.

STEP 4: Prevent Becoming Overtired

Watch for signs that your baby is becoming tired, and try to put her to bed before she gets too fussy or crying too hard to go to sleep.

STEP 5: Set a Routine

Some parents find that a routine is helpful in limiting crying episodes. Try to make your baby's schedule as predictable as possible, with feeding, bathing, sleeping, and daily outings occurring at around the same times each day.

STEP 6: Change Holding Styles

Different ways of holding the baby might help. Try using a firm hold with lots of support or hold your baby while she is swaddled tightly in a blanket. Your baby might also respond positively by being skin-to-skin with you. Try the football hold (the baby is face up, with her head supported in your hand, her back supported along your forearm, and her bottom tucked between your hip and elbow as though you were running with a football) or the colic hold (the baby is face down, with her head supported in your hand, her belly supported by and receiving pressure from your forearm while you are seated).

STEP 7: Play Music

Some families find that music or white noise is helpful. Try different types of music, turn on the vacuum or a white noise machine, or make a "shushing" noise while holding the baby over your shoulder. For some babies this noise appears to be soothing — and for some parents it drowns out the baby's cries!

STEP 8: Increase Carrying and Holding

Increased carrying and holding may help reduce the length of bouts of crying, but not the frequency. Try a baby carrier or sling if you would like to try this approach, but remember that babies get used to falling asleep under certain conditions. This extra carrying while sleeping might reduce the crying in your child now, but contribute to difficulties getting to sleep by himself later on.

STEP 9: Create Motion

Motion may reduce the crying. Slow up-and-down movements (hold the baby upright against your shoulder while doing slow knee bends) seem particularly helpful, but try other methods — jiggling gently, rocking, pushing in the stroller, going for a ride in the car, swinging in a baby swing. Just remember that your baby may become dependent on these methods to stop crying and get to sleep.

STEP 10: Maintain Eating Habits

Keep feeding your baby in the same way. It is rare for a change in eating habits to have an effect on colic. Consult your health-care provider before altering your diet or your baby's diet.

STEP 11: Limit Secondhand Smoke

Limit your baby's exposure to secondhand smoke. Babies of parents who smoke during and after pregnancy are more likely to cry excessively.

STEP 12: Improve Sleep Hygiene

If your baby's crying is always associated with trying to put her down to sleep and not just at one particular fussy time of the day, her crying may be related to her sleep and not to colic. Try following our recommendations to improve your child's sleep hygiene. For these guidelines, see Part 1, Chapter 3, "Sleep Hygiene."

Tips for Dealing with a Colicky Baby

1. **Lighten your load:** Seek some help from friends and family — don't be afraid to ask for help. If you are feeling extremely frustrated, ask someone to come and stay with the baby while you take a break. Do something, such as exercising or other physical activity, to vent your frustration or talk to a friend or family member.

2. **Get out of the house each day:** You will be better able to comfort your baby if you participate in some activities that recharge your emotional and physical energy. Join a parenting group or have someone watch the baby while you take a walk around the block. An hour to yourself each day is ideal. Being able to relax out of earshot of your crying baby is best of all, but take what you can get — even a few minutes alone in another room of the house can help.

3. **Take some time alone with your partner:** It can be easy to forget about one another when all your energy is focused on trying to soothe the baby.

4. **Never shake your baby:** This can lead to serious and permanent brain damage. If you are concerned that you are so frustrated that you might harm the baby, call a family member, your health-care provider, a crisis hotline, or even the Children's Aid Society to get help quickly.

What Is Temperamental Difference?

You may have had someone remark that your baby has a "happy," "difficult," "easy," or "fussy" temperament. Temperament is our usual mood or disposition, including our way of thinking, behaving, and reacting to situations. The characteristics that make up our temperament appear early in life and include our emotions, activity level, attention, sociability, and reactivity. For example, some children are very active, while others are more sedentary; some children readily interact with other children and adults, while others are shy; some children attend to one task for a long time, while others have an attention span that wanders quickly; and some children cry easily, while others are more easy-going.

Temperament Factors

The temperament of a child is affected by many factors. Both our genetic makeup and our environment play a role in the development of temperament, but if you have more than one biological child, do not be surprised if they each have unique temperaments.

Although your children are similar genetically and live in the same environment, there are always at least slight differences in both their genetic material and in their physical and social environments that influence their temperament. And, of course, it makes for more interesting families that we are all unique individuals!

Self-Soothing

A child's temperament in early life may predict her future emotional and social behavior in some situations, but this relationship is not so clear when it comes to behaviors surrounding bedtime and sleep. It seems logical that a more easy-going baby would be easier to put to bed and would be a more efficient sleeper, but research does not support this assumption. In fact, it seems that a more important issue is the child's ability to self-soothe. Self-soothing is the child's ability to calm himself in order to fall asleep and, upon awakening, to return to sleep without needing the presence of a parent.

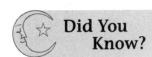
Did You Know?

Self-Soothing
Researchers have not found temperament to be linked to the ability to self-soothe, so a child who has a very easy-going temperament may not be able to self-soothe and may need a parent's presence to fall asleep.

Guidelines for Treating Temperamental Crying

Y OU CAN HELP your baby (even an infant) with increased crying and irritability by recognizing the symptoms and acting on them with behavior intervention. You can help your child learn to soothe himself at bedtime and when he wakens.

STEP 1: Recognize Tiredness

Remember that your young baby (under 6 weeks of age) will become tired after 1 to 1½ hours of being awake, and your older baby (up to 3 months of age) will become tired after being awake for 1½ to 2 hours. Look for signs of tiredness, such as frowning, decreased attention, more crying, and fussing. Put your child to sleep at these times.

STEP 2: Recognize Signs of Distress

Learn to 'read' your baby's response to stimulation. If your baby is easily startled and not able to self-soothe easily, then you may need to help him calm himself down by using a quiet and gentle approach when changing his diaper, bathing him, or settling him at sleep times.

STEP 3: Be Predictable

You can help your newborn infant transition to sleep by nursing, feeding, or rocking him. In later infancy, at least by the age of 3 months, you should establish a predictable routine of feeding and settling at naptimes and bedtime. This may be feeding, quiet play, or giving your baby a brief cuddle, then putting him in bed, drowsy but awake.

STEP 4: Remain Flexible

Your child's temperament and her sleep behaviors will change over the course of her development. You will do yourself and your child a favor by being open to those changes. Try not to develop expectations of a particular way of behaving — your baby who has trouble soothing herself to sleep might well turn into a champion sleeper as a toddler. Aim to understand more about her sleep and work to improve it.

Q. Should I take my baby to the doctor if she is crying excessively?

A. You should talk to your doctor about your baby if his crying is excessive and you or your partner is finding this problem intolerable. Even if there is no medical problem, your baby's crying may be something you cannot deal with. Your doctor can help you find a way to cope successfully.

There are signs that you should be aware of that are definite problems to discuss with your doctor:

- If your child's problems with crying do not improve by the age of 3 months
- If your baby does not respond to you when not crying, with eye contact, for example
- If your baby has other symptoms, such as excessive spitting up or vomiting with her feedings, poor weight gain, excessive straining when she has a bowel movement, skin rashes or eczema, fever, diarrhea, or other signout illness
- If your baby turns blue or seems to have trouble breathing while crying
- If there is a large change in the usual pattern of your baby's crying or activity
- If you are unable to 'bond' to your baby
- If you feel angry, anxious, depressed or have any other feelings that interfere with your ability to care for your baby

case study: **Sonja** (continued)

When a baby has persistent crying or colic like Sonja, it's important to explore contributing factors about both the baby and her parents. In this case, Maria had several pregnancy losses before Sonja was born, and she still found it hard to believe that she has a healthy, thriving infant. Regarding Sonja, she appeared to have typical colic, but her crying was increased because she was obtaining slightly less sleep for 24 hours than most 2-month-old babies and, as a result, was somewhat sleep deprived.

When Maria and Joe were able to recognize and discuss these problems, they became more relaxed about Sonja's colic. They were reassured that she would outgrow this problem, most likely by 3 to 4 months, and that her early experience with colic did not predict a difficult temperament as a child. Maria and Joe established a predictable sleep routine and used other strategies to decrease her colic. They were prepared to cope better.

Chapter 7

Confusional Arousals, Night Terrors, and Sleepwalking

I F YOU HAVE BEEN AWAKENED by your child during a night terror or sleepwalking episode, you will likely not forget it. Watching your child have a night terror is a scary experience. He may sit up abruptly in bed, let out a loud panicky scream, act in a confused and frightening way, begin to sweat with his heart racing, and look terrified. It can be equally scary to watch your child sleepwalking. Although he will not look terrified, he may walk into a dangerous situation, inside the house or outside. You are left wondering what might have happened to him if you had not woken up. To make matters worse, in both situations, if you try to soothe your child by talking to him or hugging him, he is likely to look right through you, like you are not his parent, and even get more agitated in his night terror or walking behavior.

Among sleep experts, these arousals are known as partial arousal parasomnias. Our focus in this chapter is on the three common partial arousal parasomnias: confusional arousals, night terrors, and sleepwalking. Dreams and nightmares are discussed in the next chapter.

What Are Parasomnias?

A parasomnia is a movement (sleepwalking, for example) or an experience (nightmare, for example) that occurs during sleep. Parasomnias can be part of normal sleep (dreams, for example) or abnormal (sleepwalking, for example).

Did You Know?

Arousal Timing
If your child is going to have a night terror or sleepwalking episode, it is more likely to occur within the first few hours after falling asleep during a partial waking from deep (slow-wave) NREM sleep.

Partial Arousal Parasomnias
- Confusional arousals
- Night terrors
- Sleepwalking

What are Partial Arousal Parasomnias?

A partial arousal parasomnia is an abnormal phenomenon that occurs during deep (slow-wave) NREM sleep, when your child is partially aroused from this sleep state. The majority of deep sleep is in the first third of the night.

Young children have more deep slow-wave sleep than school-age children. This deep sleep can be good for your young child (significant growth occurs during this time) or problematic (during this deep sleep your child may be partially aroused and have a night terror or sleepwalking episode). Because preschool children spend more time during sleep in this slow-wave sleep, they are more likely to have these types of arousals than older children. For more information, see Part 1, Chapter 1 "Sleep Basics."

Partial arousal parasomnias occur during an arousal from slow-wave sleep when your child is partially awake and partially asleep — sort of stuck between the two. During a partial arousal parasomnia, your child is able to carry out some activities normally associated with the waking state, like sitting up, crying out, and walking, but he is also partially asleep, so his speech will not make sense.

In these partial arousals, it is difficult to wake up fully. If you try to talk to your child or comfort him, he will not understand what you are saying, and this interaction may actually make him more agitated. He will not have normal judgment, so there is the potential to injure himself. Your child will not remember this episode in the morning.

Confusional Arousals

During this kind of partial arousal parasomnia, your child may sit up, stare with eyes open, vocalize but not scream, and appear confused. He will not likely get out of bed and walk around. The episode is usually brief, lasting a few minutes, and then he will fall back asleep.

Your child will be confused, but will not have an expression of terror characteristic to a night terror. Confusional arousals are sometimes called "sleep drunkenness."

Night Terrors

A night terror is also called a sleep terror or Pavor nocturnus. Although commonly called night terror, sleep terror is a more accurate name because the episodes can occur during daytime

Did You Know?

Amnesia
When your child is having a partial arousal, he is not dreaming and does not remember the event if not awakened from it. This experience may be very frightening to you, but will not be at all frightening to your child.

Did You Know?

Natural Tendency
Partial arousals are not a problem in childhood, but a natural tendency. These arousals are common in preschool children, but can be of concern if they persist into school age or occur for the first time in older children or adults.

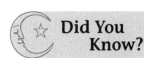

Did You Know?

Confusional Arousal Incidence
Children are most likely to experience this milder form of arousal before 5 years of age. Although we are not certain how common this arousal may be, it has been suggested that 5% to 15% of children experience confusional arousals. They rarely continue into adolescence or adulthood.

NIGHT TERROR QUESTIONNAIRE

Complete the following questionnaire if you suspect your child is experiencing night terrors.

Instructions

Check the appropriate "Y" (Yes) or "N" (No) box.

Y	N	Question
☐	☐	1. Does he awaken 1 to 3 hours after falling asleep?
☐	☐	2. Does he appear to be awake with eyes open, but does not interact with you, looking right past you as though he does not recognize you?
☐	☐	3. Does he scream violently and seem to be very frightened, with a racing heart rate, fast breathing, sweating, and dilated pupils?
☐	☐	4. If you do not try to wake him, does he fall back asleep?
☐	☐	5. Does he seem to have more arousals when he is more sleep deprived?
☐	☐	6. Does he remember this episode in the morning?

Scoring

If the answer is "Yes" to 1, 2, 3, 4, and 5, but "No" to 6, this likely means your child is experiencing night terrors. Although the answer to #6 should be 'No' when a child has a night terror, it is important to know that if you try to wake your child to stop the night terror, or talk about it to him or others in the morning, then he will remember or appear to remember what happened to him during the night. Otherwise, he will have no memory of it.

Did You Know?

Night Terror Incidence
Approximately 6% of children experience night terrors, most commonly between 2 and 4 years of age. They usually resolve within 1 to 3 years of onset, but can persist to 10 to 12 years of age. They rarely continue into adulthood.

sleep. In one of these episodes, you may find your child sitting up in bed and screaming, with a terrified facial expression in a confused state. Usually, your child will also be sweaty and breathing quickly, with a fast heart rate and dilated pupils. These are the features that are seen during the day when you are frightened. Vigorous physical activity and even violent behavior sometimes accompany night terrors. A night terror episode may be followed by sleepwalking.

You may notice that your child will be more likely to have a night terror after a stressful event or experience, or when he has had some late nights or been more sleep deprived.

Similarities and Differences Among Partial Arousal Parasomnias

Because these three sleep disturbances are all partial arousals from deep slow-wave sleep, they share many characteristics. They can be distinguished by several specific differences.

Similarities			
Behavior or Situation	**Confusional Arousal**	**Night Terror**	**Sleepwalking**
Time of night?	1 to 3 hours after falling asleep	1 to 3 hours after falling asleep	1 to 3 hours after falling asleep
Type of sleep when episode starts?	Deep slow-wave sleep	Deep slow-wave sleep	Deep slow-wave sleep
Does child awaken during episode?	No	No	No
Does child remember episode in the morning?	No	No	No
Is child confused during and after?	Yes	Yes	Yes
Does this episode occur when child is awake?	No	No	No
Is there a family history?	Common	Common	Common
Differences			
Child screams	No	Yes	No
Child walks	No	No (children can have an episode of sleepwalking after the night terror)	Yes
Duration	5 to 40 minutes	1 to 5 minutes	1 to 10 minutes
Potential for the child to harm himself	Low	Low	High
Amount of heart racing, breathing fast, sweating, pupils dilated	Moderate	Marked	Mild in calm sleepwalking to moderate in agitated sleepwalking
Amount of agitation	Moderate	Marked	None to moderate

Sleepwalking

Sleepwalking is also called somnambulism. In this episode, your child may wake up and have repetitive activity, such as picking at his bedclothes, and then get out of bed.

He will be able to walk, but will have decreased visual perception, so may trip over furniture or fall from a height and injure himself. He may also look like he is doing something purposeful, such as urinating, but may be mistaken about where the bathroom is and do so in an inappropriate place. Younger children may walk toward a light and find themselves standing quietly in your bedroom.

Causes of Partial Arousals

Partial arousals can be caused by genetic factors, deep-sleep factors, and sleep fragmenting factors.

Genetic Factors

These arousals tend to run in families. Your child may have a family member who has the same or one of the other arousal disorders.

Deep-Sleep Factors

It is natural to have more deep sleep in childhood. Some children are naturally deep sleepers. If your child has been sleep deprived and is recovering from this, he will have deeper sleep. Fever and medications, such as hypnotics and sedatives that depress the central nervous system, can also be factors in causing partial arousal parasomnias.

Sleep-Fragmenting Factors

Factors that may fragment sleep and cause an increased tendency to an arousal disturbance include:
- Stress
- Irregular sleep schedule
- Stimulant medications (which are used to treat attention deficit hyperactivity disorder)
- Stimuli in the sleep environment, such as noise or stimuli from within the body, such as pain
- Being woken from deep sleep

case study: **Daniel**

Mr. and Mrs. Brown brought their son Daniel to our sleep clinic because they were concerned about his strange behavior some nights. Daniel is a 5-year-old healthy and well-behaved boy, who happily attends kindergarten during the day. However, at night he is having episodes where he appears to be "possessed by the devil," as Mr. Brown describes his behavior.

Daniel is not always cooperative about bedtime, often fusses about going to sleep, and demands attention at night. He will finally fall asleep around 10:00 p.m., often with his father lying beside him in bed. For the past year, Daniel has been waking between 11:00 p.m. and midnight, in what appears to be a frightening dream. This happens about once a week. He sits up in bed, his pupils are dilated, his heart is racing in his chest, he is sweaty, and he screams in a "blood-curdling" manner, Mrs. Brown explains. Occasionally, this episode is followed by his getting out of bed and wandering aimlessly in the room.

During these episodes, his parents try to comfort him, but Daniel looks right through them as if they were not there. In fact, Mrs. Brown feels that her attempts to comfort him actually make his episodes worse. After about 5 minutes of this behavior, he seems to settle down, and then he quickly falls back asleep. He usually does not remember in the morning what was scaring him. Mr. and Mrs. Brown are beside themselves with worry about what is happening to their son at night….

(continued on page 167)

Guidelines for Treating Partial Arousal Parasomnias

STEP 1: Improve Sleep Hygiene

Consider the behavior factors contributing to your child's partial parasomnias, especially poor sleep hygiene and inadequate sleep. Establish a consistent sleep-wake schedule and maintain it 7 days a week. If he is having caffeinated foods or beverages, either eliminate them or do not let him have anything with caffeine for 6 hours before bedtime.

These arousals can be triggered by being awakened from a deep sleep, so make sure your child's room is quiet at night. For more guidelines for improving sleep hygiene, see Part 1, Chapter 3, "Sleep Hygiene."

STEP 2: Extend Sleep

Your child may be mildly sleep deprived, so try to encourage more sleep with an earlier bedtime.

STEP 3: Ensure Safety

Do not interfere with your child during the arousal. Watch him from a safe distance so that you can ensure his safety, especially if he gets out of bed and starts to sleepwalk. If you try to interact with a child who is having a night terror or sleepwalking, you may increase his agitation and violence. Remove furniture or objects that your child can trip on or that could be potentially harmful.

STEP 4: Let Your Child Fall Back To Sleep

Do not wake up your child. Let him finish the episode. Lead him calmly back to his bed if he got out. He will naturally fall back to sleep without your help at the end of the episode. In the morning, do not remind your child of the night terror. Do not ask him about it or describe it to him. It will be frightening for him to know that something happened during his sleep that scared his parents.

STEP 5: Reduce Sleep Fragmentation

If possible, eliminate or reduce any extraordinary stress from your child's life. A child who has a regular sleep schedule, is getting adequate sleep, and is well rested during the day, but still has frequent arousals may be under stress. The stress could be due to bullying at school, marital stress in the family, or emotional or psychological problems in your child. Consult with your doctor if you think these factors may be affecting your child's sleep behavior.

STEP 6: Treat Other Sleep Disorder Symptoms

If your child has other sleep disorders that are disturbing his sleep, this may increase the arousals. There has been some initial research showing that children with partial arousals who were treated for symptoms of obstructive sleep apnea (snoring primarily) and restless legs syndrome (with restlessness) experienced a reduction in arousal episodes. This is an area where further studies are needed. You should also talk to your health-care provider about the need for further evaluation of these problems if you think your child has signs or symptoms of other sleep disorders.

Other Treatment Options

There are other treatments sometimes recommended for treating partial arousal parasomnia. However, they have not been well studied in children or adults.

Relaxation Therapy

You may be able to decrease stress by relaxation therapy in an older child, but this is usually done under the guidance of a professional and has not been studied yet in children with arousal disorders.

Scheduled Awakenings

Some research shows that if children are woken up just before their arousal usually occurs, then allowed to fall back asleep, this may change the child's sleep state and decrease the arousals. This strategy could only be used if your child has a consistent time for the arousal to occur. It has not been well studied, so we don't know if it is really an effective treatment.

Medication

Some doctors use medications to try and 'break the cycle' for a child with a very frequent arousal disorder. Medications would only be used after all of the causes of arousals have been reviewed and eliminated. Medication does not 'stop' or 'cure' the arousals, but may be helpful to change the pattern of sleep temporarily. We don't know for sure who should be tried on medications. When children are seen with arousal disorders, it is very rare to consider this option.

SAFETY FOR SLEEPWALKERS

It is very important to consider safety measures if your child sleepwalks. He could definitely harm himself when sleepwalking because he is able to walk, but is not fully aware of where he is going and has decreased ability to maneuver around objects. These are some of the suggestions for your sleepwalker.

- Do not sleep in the top bunk.

- Clear the bedroom of obstacles that he can trip over.

- Put alarms or locks on doors to balconies, the basement, the kitchen or other rooms with dangerous objects.

- Put an alarm on the bedroom door, so that you will know if he leaves the bedroom.

- Be especially cautious when your child sleeps at a friend's house or when you are traveling and staying in an unfamiliar accommodation that has not been safety proofed for a sleepwalker.

Q. When should I be concerned about my child and discuss his arousals with my doctor?

A. Remember that these episodes are seen in healthy, normal children at a young age and most outgrow them by 10 years of age. However, if any of the following situations arise, contact your doctor.

- If the arousals (especially night terrors) start after the age of 7 years

- If the arousal does not occur in the first 1 to 3 hours after falling asleep

- If the arousals are frequent or increasing in frequency or duration despite trying to eliminate the causes as discussed in this chapter.

- If the arousals are accompanied by other unusual behavior, such as self-injury, or your child has signs of another sleep disorder, such as bed-wetting or sleep apnea with snoring or pauses in breathing

- If your child remembers the event in the morning, especially if you don't wake him from the arousal

- If your child is tired the following day

- If there is anything about the arousal that makes you consider that it is a seizure or a 'fit'. This would include repetitive or rhythmic behavior, movements during the beginning of the arousal that look the same every night, episodes where the child sustains any injuries, or experiences daytime fatigue

- If you suspect other problems in your child, such as emotional upset, anxiety, excessive stress, bullying at school, or any similar difficulties

case study: **Daniel** (continued)

We determined that Daniel was probably somewhat sleep deprived because his parents were having problems with bedtime settling, and at the age of 5 years, he was falling asleep at 10:00 p.m. In children who are prone to have night terrors, inadequate sleep is a common factor, which increases the frequency of the episodes. Although they are a normal developmental phenomenon and can occur in well-rested children, night terrors are precipitated by an irregular sleep schedule.

Daniel's parents were relieved to learn that their son's nighttime behavior was a common occurrence in young children and was not associated with any long-lasting behavior, personality, or psychiatric disorders. Mr. and Mrs. Brown made two major changes, which they felt were helpful in resolving the night terrors. First, they learned more about limit setting and developed a more consistent sleep routine. They set limits about bedtime, so that over time, Daniel began to be more agreeable at bedtime and was soon falling asleep at 9:00 instead of 10:00 p.m. Second, they changed their pattern of responding to him when he had a night terror. They watched him from across the room to make sure that he did not harm himself. Although they found it very hard not to try to comfort Daniel when he seemed so frightened and confused, it actually made the night terrors shorter when they did not interfere. This way, they could see that Daniel finished the night terror and then went back to sleep. He then slept peacefully until the morning.

The Browns noticed that over the next few years, the night terrors became less frequent, and by the age of 7, Daniel stopped having them altogether. They were happy about this, but are a bit worried about their infant, Jenny, and when (or if) she is also going to develop the same problem.

Chapter 8

Nightmares and Nighttime Anxiety

H AVING A NIGHTMARE is an experience we can all relate to. You wake up with a sense of dread and fear, sometimes with the sensation that you are unable to breathe or move. Soon after waking, an adult will become alert enough to realize he has had a nightmare and will be able to return to sleep. However, for a child, especially a young child, this will be an even more frightening experience because a child may have difficulty differentiating a nightmare from reality. A child will be more likely to get frightened when woken from a nightmare and have more difficulty returning to sleep. You cannot abolish all nightmares in your child, but you can learn more about them, and the steps to take to decrease their frequency.

Nighttime anxiety is a different problem from nightmares, but is included in this chapter because you need to learn how to differentiate what is preventing your child from peaceful sleep. Is it anxiety about going to sleep due to the possibility of a nightmare, or is your child generally anxious and his anxiety is more obvious at night? If your child has general anxiety, you can help him by reading this chapter and gaining an understanding of how to decrease his anxiety around sleep, but he probably also needs to be evaluated by your health-care provider for other general strategies or treatment for anxiety.

What Are Nightmares?

A nightmare (which is also called a dream anxiety attack) is a dream with frightening content. Nightmares, like dreams, probably occur in all stages of sleep, but you only can remember them when you wake from a nightmare in REM (which is typically considered to be dreaming sleep).

During REM sleep, your brain waves look similar to their pattern during waking, which indicates that during this sleep stage our minds are active and thought to be forming memories. You are also more easily fully aroused during this state. This is

Did You Know?

First Nightmares
Nightmares most frequently occur in the preschool years. We don't really know at what age you can start to experience a nightmare, but infants spend 50% of their sleep time in REM sleep, so it is possible that they could have nightmares. However, we would not know until children have enough language to describe a nightmare, which would typically not be before 2 years of age.

why you can remember your dreams and nightmares when you wake from this state.

During REM sleep, your muscles (except those muscles responsible for eye movements, hearing, and breathing) have less tone and are more floppy, which is why you may experience a feeling of fright when you wake up. You may know at some level of consciousness that you are scared and in trouble during a nightmare, but you can't react or move away from whatever is frightening you.

The occurrence of nightmares remains frequent until about age 10 years of age, and then they become less common. However, as most people know, they continue occasionally throughout life.

Characteristics of Nightmares

General Characteristics

- Nightmares happen in the early morning hours when you have longer and more frequent periods of REM sleep.

- During nightmares, you may have a feeling of agonizing dread, with a sense of weight on your chest, which feels like it is interfering with your ability to breath.

- While waking from a nightmare, you may have the experience of feeling briefly paralyzed.

- When you wake up, you may have a fast heart rate, be breathing quickly, and feel sweaty.

Characteristics of Children's Nightmares

- When your child awakes from a nightmare, he will be fully aroused, oriented to his environment, and able to speak clearly because the threshold to waking from REM sleep is low, unlike in a night terror, when he awakes only partially from deep sleep.

- Upon waking from a nightmare, your child will likely still have signs of anxiety, but he will respond to being comforted by you. He will be fully aware of your presence.

- After a nightmare, your child may be able to clearly recall the content of the nightmare. The content of the nightmare will be appropriate to the developmental level of your child. For example, a young child may be afraid of dogs and monsters, while an adolescent may be afraid of something he saw in the movies or a more realistic fear of an event he read about or saw reported on television.

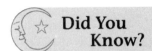

Did You Know?

Nightmare Incidence
Nightmares are most frequent between the ages of 3 and 6. During these ages, young children have more fears (both during the day and at night) because they are not always clear about what is imaginary and what is real. Nightmares also commonly occur in later childhood. In a study of healthy children between 5 and 12 years, 30% had experienced at least one nightmare in the last 6 months. Problematic nightmares, defined as a problem lasting more than 3 months, were present in 24% of children ages 2 to 5 years, 41% of children ages 6 to 10 years, and in 22% of children age 11 years.

Drug Causes of Nightmares
- Some antidepressants
- Some benzodiazepines
- Beta blockers
- Withdrawal from alcohol, barbiturates, or benzodiazepines

Causes of Nightmares

Fever, stress, or any factor that causes sleep deprivation, such as an irregular sleep schedule, can cause nightmares, a well as any sleep disorder that disrupts sleep, such as sleep apnea. Taking some medications is associated with nightmares as is withdrawal from some medications.

Folk Treatments for Frequent Nightmares

Some people recommend that you help the child to feel safe by spraying the room with anti-monster water, for example, or by checking under the beds to make sure there are no monsters. Others say not to do this because it confuses the child about what is real and what is fantasy. What is recommended?

There is no science to recommend for or against either of these methods. We don't know if one method increases or decreases nightmares as compared to the other. You need to use your own judgment to decide how to decrease the anxiety in your own child.

case history: Jennifer

Jennifer is a 5-year-old girl whose parent brought her to our sleep clinic because of frequent nightmares. These started 2 months ago after her house was robbed. Although Jennifer and her family were not home at the time, they returned to see that the house had been ransacked. Jennifer was very aware of both her parents' distress.

Shortly after the incident, she began to wake from sleep two to three times per week, usually around 3:00 a.m., and seemed to be reliving the robbery. Her parents had tried to show her that the house had new locks and was safe, but this hadn't yet seemed to help....

(continued on page 172)

Guidelines for Treating Nightmares

ALTHOUGH NIGHTMARES ARE a common problem, there has been very little research about the treatment of nightmares in children. These are our recommendations for children who have frequent nightmares. If the nightmares are persistent, consider further evaluation by your health-care provider for other stresses or anxiety that may be contributing factors.

STEP 1: Avoid Sleep Deprivation

Avoid sleep deprivation, which can trigger nightmares. Avoid foods that lead to decreased sleep, like caffeinated foods and beverages. For more guidelines for improving sleep hygiene, see Part 1, Chapter 3, "Sleep Hygiene."

STEP 2: Decrease Exposure to Frightening Information

To decrease the frequency of nightmares, think about what your child is exposed to that may be triggering the events. This will change depending on his age and level of development. For a young child, curtail his exposure to violence in video games, television programs, cartoons, and movies. In addition to these activities, an older child may be exposed to frightening or violent material in the news media, in books, or even in discussions that he hears at home or in the community.

STEP 3: Respond Positively

When your child has a nightmare, minimize your own anxiety about the nightmare. The less you react in a scared way, the better. Respond to your child's needs. Make sure he knows that he is safe and that you will protect him. If your child is able and willing to speak, ask him to describe what is frightening. Then explain that this is a bad dream and is not real.

STEP 4: Use a Security Object

Encourage your child to have a security object — a special blanket or stuffed animal, for example — that he associates with falling asleep at bedtime. This may help him to fall back asleep more quickly after the occurrence of a nightmare.

STEP 5: Wind Down

Leave your child's bedroom after the nightmare occurs when he is calm and not awake. Try not to bring him into your bed, which will increase the attention he receives and may increase the frequency of nightmares. You can leave a night-light on during the night.

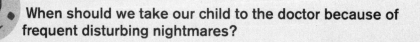

Q. When should we take our child to the doctor because of frequent disturbing nightmares?

A. See your doctor if your child's nightmare and sleep behavior take on these characteristics:

- If your child's nightmares are persistent or frequent

- If the nightmares are affecting your child's ability to function during the day

- If the nightmares are causing the development of secondary bedtime fears

- If the nightmares are related to disturbing content (abuse or trauma, for example)

---

case study: **Jennifer** (continued)

Jennifer's nightmares remained frequent for the first 6 months following the home robbery. When her parents came to the clinic to talk about these nightmares, they explained that after each nightmare, she had been allowed to sleep between them in the parental bedroom.

We recommended changing this behavior. Now, Jennifer's parents go to their daughter's room after each nightmare and calm her down, but then insist that she stay in her room to fall asleep. Because she did not want to do this initially, her parents agreed to sit in a chair beside her bed until she fell asleep. They were about to start a chair-sitting routine, where they would gradually withdraw from her bed slowly at the time of the nightmare, but, unexpectedly, the nightmares seemed to resolve on their own.

Jennifer still has occasional nightmares, but once she is reassured by one of her parents, she is able to fall back asleep in her own bed. We expect her nightmares will resolve with time.

What Are Nighttime Fears?

Nighttime fears are very common during childhood and occur at bedtime or upon waking during the night. During the day, it is easier for your child to keep worrisome thoughts at bay because she is generally active and occupied with play. At night, when your child has more opportunity to be quiet and think, anxieties may rise to the surface. As your child gets sleepy, frightening thoughts may come to the surface, and she has less control over her feelings.

Developmental Stages

Most children experience nighttime fears at some point in their development, but they express different fears at different ages and developmental stages.

Infants: Separation Anxiety

At about 6 months of age, babies realize that you are a separate person, and in the next few months, they learn that you still exist when you are out of their sight. They may fear that you will not return to them once you have gone. Before children are comfortable with the idea that you have not left them alone permanently, separation anxiety is very common, especially at night.

Preschoolers: Imaginary Things and Events

Preschoolers become frightened of imaginary things or events, frightening creatures, and the dark. The most common age for bedtime fears is 3 to 6 years of age.

Older Children: Natural Disasters and Supernatural Phenomena

Older children develop fears of more realistic life situations or natural disasters, such as tornadoes or floods, as well as supernatural phenomena, such as ghosts.

Adolescents: School Performance and Social Situations

Adolescents experience anxiety at night related to future events and concerns about their performance at school or problems with social situations, in addition to other fears.

Nighttime Fear or Sleep Delay Tactic?

Some children manipulate nighttime fears to delay going to sleep. How will you recognize a fearful child from one who realizes that expressing fears at bedtime is a way to delay going to sleep? Check out this chart.

Fearful child	Child stalling to delay going to sleep
May revert to more childlike, immature behavior at night	Level of maturity will be the same during the day as at night
May cry, be clingy, and resist going to bed	Will not display other behaviors indicating fear at night, such as crying, clinging
Will be comforted at night by having you in the room and demands will cease	Will have many demands — "I want you in the room, I want more water…more stories…"
Will likely display fear during the day — will not separate to attend day care, school, play with friends	Will not show fear or anxiety during the day — will separate and attend activities with minimal or no problems
Will display similar behavior during the day, which worsens at night	Nighttime fears will be unexpected from daytime behavior

Guidelines for Treating Nighttime Fears

STEP 1: Establish a Relaxing Bedtime Routine and Environment

This is especially important for a child who tends to be anxious. A brief, enjoyable routine, such as a healthy snack, brushing teeth, and a quiet story, can help your child to relax. If your child is afraid of the dark, it may be helpful to use a night-light or leave her door open to the rest of the house when she goes to bed. If your child is having trouble being alone in her room at nighttime, she may benefit from doing fun activities in her bedroom during the day. For more guidelines on establishing a relaxing bedtime routine and sleep environment, see Part 1, Chapter 3, "Sleep Hygiene."

STEP 2: Reduce Evening Stimulation

Reducing stimulating activities before bedtime can reduce nighttime anxiety.

1. Avoid television programs, movies, and computer games that depict frightening scenes, including nighttime news programs. Although it may seem that your child is not paying attention, engrossed in his own play world, he can still absorb disturbing details on the news.

2. Avoid roughhousing and vigorous play at bedtime. Children should be quietly winding down in the time before they go to bed. Read bedtime stories that are calm in nature and have happy endings. Avoid stories that involve cliff-hangers or sad endings.

STEP 3: Address the Fear

If your child has certain fears that need to be addressed, discuss the details of what your child is afraid of during the daytime hours. Avoid discussing difficult or frightening topics with your child or having such discussions with your partner around your child during the hours leading up to bedtime. Discussing nighttime fears right before going to bed can exacerbate the anxiety. Talk to your child about her fears and other ways to respond to the fears than crying and calling out for you.

STEP 4: Calm the Fear of Separation

Let your child see you walk out the bedroom door as this helps them learn to tolerate separation from you – do not sneak out. If your child has seen you leave and has been reassured that you are still in the house to care for him, he will not wonder if you are really at home and will trust that you will be there for him.

STEP 5: Think Positively

Talk about what might work to make the fears go away, such as saying positive self-statements like "I am brave" and "Monsters are not real." You might try reading a children's storybook about a character who learns to overcome her bedtime fears. 'Searching' your child's room for 'monsters' may send the message that indeed there are monsters in her room. If your child expresses fears of scary creatures, explain to her in a matter-of-fact way that monsters do not exist.

STEP 6: Reassure Your Child

Reassure your child and communicate to her that she is safe.

1 Let her know that you are close by to her and will make sure that nothing bad happens to her. For example, tell her, "Mummy and Daddy are right downstairs and we'll always make sure that you are safe."

2 Some families like to use a checking schedule at bedtime. If your child knows that every 10 minutes or so one parent will check in on her, she may be able to relax and fall asleep knowing that your presence is reliable.

3 If your child wakes up in the middle of the night with fear, go to her bedroom and reassure her there. If she comes to your room, get right up and return her to her bedroom and reassure her in her own room.

4 Avoid bringing your child into bed with you to calm her fears or to sleep with you. You do not want to give positive reinforcement for your child's fear-related behavior and thereby create habits, which are hard to break. You must set firm and consistent limits so that your child stays in her bedroom and limits her crying and calling out to you. If these problems continue, she may become dependent on your attention to fall asleep, so you need to be firm and consistent in your approach.

STEP 7: Reward Appropriate Bedtime Behavior

Some children respond very well to a reward system for appropriate bedtime behavior. For example, your child could receive a gold star on a calendar for each day she remains in her room or for each night she doesn't call out for you once in bed. The stars can then be traded in for a reward that is meaningful to your child. The behaviors required to receive the rewards should be as specific as possible — not a star for being "good," but a star for "staying in your bed all night."

STEP 8: Develop Coping Skills

Older children can be taught coping skills to deal with their nighttime fears. Relaxation strategies, such as deep breathing, can help children relieve their anxiety at nighttime and make the transition to sleep. Visual imagery may be helpful as well. Instead of the fearful situations she is imagining, your child can envision herself engaging in enjoyable activities, at a favorite location, or with her best friend.

Tips for Reducing Nighttime Fears

1 **Establish safety procedures:** Occasionally, children's nighttime fears develop from events in their lives. If your child is fearful of intruders because your neighbors had their house broken into, it is important to address these issues in a reassuring manner. Depending on the age of the child, you might review the safety procedures within your home, such as fire escape routes, and how to make an emergency call to the police, fire department, and ambulance service.

2 **Offer sibling or pet comfort:** Let your child sleep with a sibling in the room, with limits set on not disrupting the sibling's sleep. If you have a pet, you can have a trial of letting the pet sleep in your child's room to determine if this decreases nighttime anxiety.

3 **Open the parental bedroom:** You can temporarily have your child sleep in the parental room (perhaps with a mattress on the floor beside you) or you can sleep in his room until the fears are conquered.

Q. When should we contact our doctor about our child's nighttime fears?

A. Some children's anxiety is severe and should be addressed by a health-care professional who deals with anxiety-related problems. If your child has generalized anxiety and it seems worse at night, then your child may have an anxiety disorder, rather than a sleep disorder. Contact your health-care provider for help if your anxious child shows these signs:

- If your child's bedtime fears are persistent and severe and don't respond to the strategies suggested in this chapter

- If the fears have been triggered by a traumatic event (for example, a robbery at your home) and become more intense over time, instead of fading as expected

- If your child's nighttime fears are accompanied by panic and your attempts to be firm and set limits lead to increasing his panic

- If your child's fears and anxiety are also present during the day and interfere with daily routine or activities

- If there is a family history of anxiety disorders

- If your child displays signs of a panic attack, such as shortness of breath, faintness, racing heart, nausea, choking sensation, chest pain, fear of losing control, or even dying

Chapter 9

Snoring, Apnea, and Hypoventilation

ONE OF THE MOST RELAXING parts of your day may be when you finish your household tasks in the evening, you have tucked your children into bed, and you have some time to yourself or to enjoy with your partner. You kick back, ready to enjoy a quiet evening — and then you hear your child snoring. If you have a child who snores, you won't be able to relax even when she is sleeping. That adult-sounding noise she is making will leave you disturbed and puzzled, even if your child is sleeping soundly.

Even more puzzling and disturbing is to watch your child stop breathing momentarily when she is sleeping. You may have already noticed that her breathing pattern is not completely regular, broken up with short pauses. Sometimes these pauses are just a part of a normal pattern, but if the pauses are long enough and the breathing is very irregular, this may be a sign of a problem called central sleep apnea or obstructive sleep apnea syndrome.

Another, less common, type of breathing problem in sleep is called hypoventilation. A child who hypoventilates during sleep breathes too infrequently or her breaths are too small, so she is not providing her body with enough oxygen.

COMMON SLEEP BREATHING PROBLEMS

- Snoring: noisy sounds your child makes during sleep from the partial collapse of the airway, causing vibration of the tissues of the airway.

- Apnea: pauses in your child's breathing (sometimes for what seems an alarmingly long time), during which he does not seem to be making any attempt to breathe, or pauses when he seems to have difficulty breathing, apparently struggling for breath, again while making no noise.

- Hypoventilation: when your child is breathing either shallowly or taking small or infrequent breaths.

Breathing Process

To understand breathing problems in sleep, let's look at what is involved in your child's normal breathing process. Breathing involves breathing in and breathing out.

Breathing In

Breathing in requires muscle work. When you breathe in, the breathing muscles (the diaphragm, the muscle between the chest and the tummy) and the intercostals (the muscles that run between the ribs) contract, expanding the chest. This creates a negative pressure, effectively acting like a vacuum cleaner, sucking air into the lungs. Because the throat is floppy, the muscles of the tongue and at the base of the throat need to hold it open; otherwise, the throat would collapse every time we breathed in.

Breathing Out

Breathing out usually requires no muscle effort because the lungs and chest are elastic, just like a balloon. Breathing out occurs simply by relaxing the breathing muscles, creating a positive pressure in the chest, allowing you to exhale. This pressure will also keep the throat open, even without any muscle effort.

Conscious and Unconscious Brain Control

This whole, complex process is controlled by a very small area situated at the base of the brain, where the brain joins the spinal cord, called the brain stem. The actual part of the brain controlling this process (think of this like having a computer chip that controls breathing) is called the respiratory nuclei. This is a subconscious part of the brain, controlling things we do without even thinking about them.

When you are awake, a number of other areas within the brain, including the conscious part of the brain, called the frontal lobes (situated just behind the eyes), also control your breathing, such as when you are talking, blowing bubbles, or swallowing. When you go to sleep, these areas also go to sleep, leaving the brain stem alone to control breathing. If there is damage to the brain stem or if it does not work properly, your child may breathe fine while awake, but have apnea while sleeping.

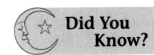

Did You Know?

Breathing Problems
Several factors can increase the chance of breathing problems, including the size of your child's tonsils and adenoids, problems with growth of the bones in the middle of the face, inflammation of the lining of the nose from allergies (called allergic rhinitis), obesity, and a decrease of muscle tone (floppiness) in the upper airway.

BREATHING PROBLEM SITES

To understand breathing problems better, consider how our airways function. If you imagine that the person in this illustration is breathing air in through his nose, marked by the arrow, you will see there are three sites it passes on its way down to the lungs: (A) the upper area above the soft palate; (B) the middle area at the level of the tonsils and adenoids; and (C) the lower area above the voice box. These sites are divided by the dotted lines.

The upper portion (A) comprises the nose and hard palate, which are rigid, encased in bone. The lower portion (C) comprises the voice box and windpipe, which are likewise rigid, made of cartilage. However, the middle portion, comprising the tongue, soft palate, and throat, is floppy to enable you to swallow and talk. You can think of these three areas as being like a vacuum cleaner hose, with a floppy portion in the middle and rigid hose on either side.

Obstruction during sleep can occur at any of these areas, but collapse of the airway during sleep is most likely to occur at area B, being the floppiest and most dependent upon muscle tone to stay open.

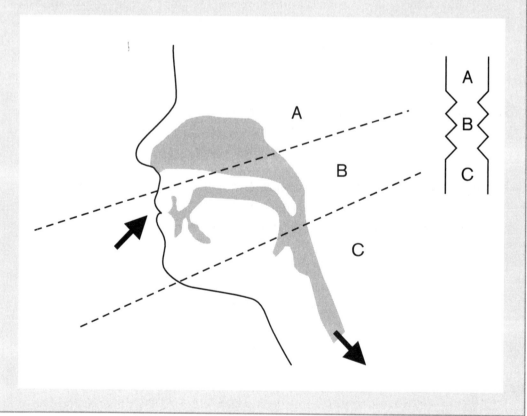

How Are Breathing Problems in Sleep Evaluated?

To determine the type and severity of breathing problems in sleep, medical professionals may conduct these evaluation procedures:

- Medical history: This will include asking if your child has signs of disturbed sleep or breathing problems during sleep.
- Sleep apnea diary: Keeping a sleep apnea diary is a helpful tool you can use when explaining to your doctor what you are observing in your child's breathing at night.
- Lateral X-ray of face: This helps to see the size of your child's adenoids and the spaces in the breathing passages.
- Overnight oximetry: Your doctor may arrange for your child to wear a sticker or probe on his finger to measure his oxygen level while he is sleeping.
- Polysomnography: This sleep study is conducted in a special sleep laboratory, using a polygraph to make a continuous record during sleep of multiple physiological variables (such as breathing, heart rate, and muscle activity).

SLEEP APNEA DIARY

If you think that your child has problems with his breathing during sleep, you need to give your health-care provider a good description of what exactly happens when your child stops breathing at night. Try keeping a sleep apnea diary that answers the following questions based on your observations. If your child has frequent and repeated episodes, making a video of several of these episodes is extremely valuable to help the health-care provider decide whether any further tests are necessary.

Q. What time of night do the apnea episodes occur?

A. _____

_____

Q. Was my child making any unusual movements or sounds before or during the episode?

A. _____

_____

Q. Did my child seem to be struggling to breathe during the episode or was he lying quietly, without any evidence of trying to breathe?

A. _____

_____

Q. How long did the episode last? You should count slowly or use a watch to try and get an accurate idea of how long the episode lasted. (When you're worried about your child's breathing, time can seem very drawn out and you may think that the episode is longer than it really is.)

A. _____

_____

Q. Is there any change in your child's skin color or appearance? What changes in color occur during the episode? Turn on the bedroom light first to assess his color and then wake up the child if necessary. (See caution below.)

A. _____

_____

Caution: If there is any change in the child's color to either blue or pale in complexion, this is not normal, and the child should be woken up. If there is no change in the child's color, it is safe to wait for 15 to 20 seconds, simply to see if your child is going to start breathing again on her own. The child may have a bluish tinge in the skin around the mouth or fingers, yet the tongue and conjunctivae (the white part of the eyeball and inside lining of the eyelids) are not. This usually occurs because of poor circulation, such as when your child is 'blue with cold,' rather than cyanosis (low oxygen in the blood).

Sleep Study

If your health-care provider suspects that your child is experiencing a significant sleep problem, your child may be referred to a sleep clinic for a sleep study. A sleep study (polysomnography) is performed in a special laboratory (sleep laboratory), either in a hospital or community laboratory. A sleep study is a noninvasive test, meaning that no needles are used, and there are actually no risks involved.

A variety of stick-on electronic sensors are used to measure your child's sleep level. Small electrodes placed on the scalp measure the electrical activity of the brain. Electrodes on both sides of the eyes and under the chin measure movement of the eyes and muscle tone. Belts are placed around the chest and tummy to measure the breathing pattern of your child. A small tube may also be placed under your child's nose to measure the air moving as he breathes. More electrodes may also be glued to your child's legs to measure how restless he is while sleeping.

The amount of oxygen in your child's blood can be measured without using needles by a machine called a pulse oximeter. It measures oxygen level simply by shining a combination of red and blue lights on a finger or toe. Because blood-containing oxygen is red while blood without oxygen is blue, the amount of red and blue light absorbed by the finger or toe can tell health-care professionals how much oxygen is in the blood.

Although a sleep study seems somewhat elaborate, it is not risky, and your child will usually be able to settle to sleep. All of these sensors are required to measure not only your child's breathing, but also if there is any disturbance in your child's sleep.

case study: **Kevin**

Anne is a 36-year-old single mother who brought her son, Kevin, to our clinic with concerns about his breathing problems at night. Kevin is 5 years old, tall and thin. His mother is worried that he snores too loudly, and she explains that this has been happening for the past 2 years.

At first, Anne thought he was only snoring when he had a cold, but recently she noticed that he is snoring almost every night. She thought that she could continue to tolerate his snoring by closing his door and hers, but a few weeks ago when there were guests staying in the home, Anne shared her bed with Kevin and noticed that he also stopped breathing for what seemed like several minutes.

Since that night, Anne has kept Kevin in her bed so she can watch him. She is exhausted from watching his breathing pauses, but is so worried about him that she can't go to sleep herself. She notices that after the pauses, Kevin will give a little snort, then seem to wake briefly and then fall back asleep. In passing, Anne also mentions that Kevin seems to be very happy in his morning kindergarten class, but he is having difficulty paying attention and cooperating in afternoon day care.

Anne is not sure what to do. She wants to know if this is the way children breathe or if Kevin has a problem. She also wants to know if she can sleep at night, or if something will happen to Kevin if she doesn't watch him....

(continued on page 189)

What Is Sleep Apnea?

Partial collapse of the airway during sleep will cause vibration of the tissues of the airway, resulting in snoring. Because you can hear a noise, there is still air flowing through the throat, so this is not apnea. If the airway closes off completely, there is no airflow and therefore no noise. This is called obstructive sleep apnea syndrome (OSAS).

Apnea is defined as an absence of any effective breathing or airflow into the lungs, usually for at least 10 seconds (in older children), or at least three missed breaths (in younger children). There are three different types of sleep apnea, each with varying degrees of severity. Central sleep apnea, which may cause brief pauses in breathing during certain sleep, can be normal or may be significant, needing evaluation. Obstructive sleep apnea, which causes episodes of prolonged partial or complete airway obstruction, may signify a major problem that needs to be investigated and treated. Mixed pattern sleep apnea, which has elements of both central and obstructive apnea, also needs to be investigated and treated.

If your child is otherwise completely well, growing and thriving, alert and happy during the day, and doing well in school without evidence of sleep disturbance other than the apnea, there is not likely to be anything significantly wrong. If, however, you have further concerns, you should consult with your health-care provider.

Central Sleep Apnea

Central sleep apnea (CSA) means that the child is making no attempt to breathe, almost as if he has forgotten to breathe. The child lies quietly, without evidence of any attempt at breathing. Central sleep apnea of less than 20 seconds (and even up to 30 seconds), if there are no other symptoms or changes in your child, is rarely associated with any significant disease or disorder.

The biggest difference between central (no attempt at breathing) and obstructive (trying to breathe through an obstructed airway) sleep apnea is simply whether the child is making an effort to breathe during the episode. However, this can be difficult to distinguish, especially if the child also snores.

Possible Associated Conditions

Usually, there are other clear signs to warn you that the child has some other illness. For example, gastroesophageal reflux (which causes heartburn), if it occurs during sleep, can result in central apnea. The child also may also have choking episodes during

 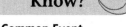

sleep, complain of heartburn, or even vomit. Seizures can also present with central apnea, but in association with odd repetitive movements during sleep, as well as self-injury during the event, and daytime fatigue. There may also be other neurological symptoms during the day. If you think that your child has symptoms of these problems, you should discuss this with your doctor.

Obstructive Sleep Apnea Syndrome

During sleep, the muscles of the throat tend to relax, particularly during REM sleep when your muscles are relaxed and with decreased tone, except for your diaphragm, hearing, and eye muscles. The throat muscles are at risk of collapsing during inspiration (drawing air into the lungs). If there is either narrowing of the airway (due to large adenoids, for example) or if the tissues of the airway are unusually floppy (due to the child being overweight), then the airway may tend to collapse during inspiration. If your child has OSAS, his sleep will be disturbed by the frequent waking episodes at night, even if the episodes don't last long enough for him to remember the episodes in the morning.

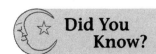

Did You Know?

Prevalence of Snoring and OSAS
About 8% to 12% of children snore most nights, while OSAS is present in 1% to 2% of children. The loudness of your child's snoring does not always relate to the amount of upper airway obstruction. He may be very loud with little obstruction or have quiet snoring with significant obstruction.

OBSTRUCTIVE SLEEP APNEA SYNDROME SYMPTOMS

To determine if your child is experiencing obstructive sleep apnea syndrome, look for these symptoms:

- Your child will look like he is struggling to breathe during sleep, but without any sound of breathing.

- If the airways are obstructed, your child can do one of two things, either try to breathe harder (which will only make the obstruction worse) or wake up. There are very powerful signals to wake up, triggered if she is having trouble breathing during sleep. Most children wake up very quickly if their airway gets obstructed.

- As soon as the child wakes up, muscle tone returns to normal, which then opens up the throat, relieving the obstruction.

- Your child will usually go right back to sleep, although some children do wake up and even get out of bed. Either way, this results in disturbed sleep.

- Your child may sweat during sleep.

- Your child may try to sleep in an unusual position in an attempt to keep his air passages open.

- The next day your child may experience memory, learning, behavioral, irritability, attention, or daytime fatigue problems.

Although many parents fear this may cause death, it is extremely rare from OSAS, chiefly because any normal child, if experiencing difficulty breathing during sleep, will wake up. They then usually take several deep breaths and go right back to sleep.

These repeated awakenings will, however, result in disrupted sleep. Consequently, your child may have difficulty with memory, learning, behavior, irritability, attention, or daytime fatigue as a consequence of obstructive sleep apnea.

OSAS Causes in Adults and Children

The causes of OSAS are different in children than in adults. The majority of adults with OSAS are overweight or obese, whereas most children are not. Unfortunately, because of the increasing number of overweight children, there are more and more children with 'adult type' OSAS.

The majority of adults with OSAS are males, but girls and boys before puberty are equally likely to be affected. Large adenoids and tonsils are only related to OSAS in children.

Another cause of OSAS in children is allergies if there is also obstruction to the breathing passages. In addition, children with any medical problem that causes narrowing of the upper airways, more floppy muscle tone, or those who have damage to their brain stem (the area of the brain controlling breathing) are at increased risk of OSAS.

Mixed Pattern Sleep Apnea

In this mixed pattern, the child usually starts off with a central apnea, but at the end of the central apnea, although the child tries to breathe, he does not open up his throat enough, and the apnea then evolves into an obstructive pattern.

Guidelines for Treating Sleep Apnea

Central Sleep Apnea

If the central sleep apnea episodes are normal physiologic events, no treatment is necessary. If they reflect an underlying disease, then treatment needs to be aimed specifically at that problem. If you suspect the problem results from another condition, you need to consult with your health-care provider and follow her guidelines for treatment.

Obstructive Sleep Apnea Syndrome

Treatment of OSAS depends on the severity of the child's apnea, ranging from a nuisance (snoring without any significant impact on sleep), through mild to moderate (causing sleep disturbance with deterioration in daytime functioning) to life threatening (a child who is unable to breath at all during sleep, resulting in recurrent, protracted episodes of apnea while the child tries to get some sleep).

STEP 1: Reduce Weight

Children who are overweight are significantly more likely to develop obstructive sleep apnea syndrome than other children. Although being overweight may not be the primary cause, it may be the tipping point because fat tissue does not accumulate simply on the tummy, but also around the neck, both narrowing the throat and making it more floppy. If your child is significantly overweight, even relatively small amounts of weight loss can have a significant impact. Weight management is advisable for improving the child's overall health. Consult with your health-care provider about strategies for helping your child with weight loss.

STEP 2: Stop Smoking

Obstructive sleep apnea is significantly more likely in children whose parents smoke. In this situation, simply not exposing children to secondhand smoke may have a significant impact. Nothing else may be required. Since cigarette smoke is a gas and spreads readily throughout the house, this means that all smoking should occur outside, where children are not as easily exposed to the gas.

STEP 3: Try Medications

Your doctor may give your child a trial of topical steroids, which can be prescribed as a nasal spray. Any chronic irritation, such as hay fever or persistent exposure to secondhand smoke, will result in swelling of the nose lining and produce obstruction. Corticosteroids are a group of compounds that reduce inflammation (different from the steroids that athletes use to build muscle). A nasal spray containing topical steroids (which are poorly absorbed, only working on the nose lining, and thus having minimal to no side effects) may help alleviate the obstructive sleep apnea. Most children, however, find it difficult to be taking these medicines for a long term, so this treatment usually can only be used for relatively short periods (such as the hay fever season).

STEP 4: Consider Surgery

There are different surgical options, but the majority of children with OSAS have their adenoids and tonsils removed to resolve the problem.

Adenotonsillectomy: Although large adenoids and tonsils may not be the primary cause of the obstructive sleep apnea, they may be the final trigger, resulting in a narrow or an excessively floppy airway. Provided their nose is not obstructed by large adenoids, most children are able to breathe adequately. However, if their airway is already narrow or excessively floppy and their adenoids become enlarged, they may obstruct the back of their nose, sufficient to cause obstructive sleep apnea.

About 90% of children with OSAS will be entirely cured or significantly improve when their adenoids and tonsils are removed. Most surgeons will remove a child's tonsils and adenoids at the same time; however, the research is mixed about whether the problem can be resolved by just taking out the adenoids.

Taking out adenoids and tonsils in children with OSAS may decrease the problems that they have with behavior and learning caused by disrupted sleep. Currently, there is a lot of scientific interest in the relationship between these problems. For the most up-to-date information, you should ask your doctor about new studies in this area.

Facial surgery: Some children may be born with abnormalities in the structure of their face, resulting in either a small upper jaw (the maxilla) or lower jaw (mandible). This can result in the narrowing of the child's airway, putting the child at risk of obstructive sleep apnea syndrome. Sometimes, with growth, this problem will cure itself. If it persists, however, the child will need surgery to correct this problem. Usually the ideal timeframe is to delay surgery until the child's face has at least partially, if not fully, grown, often after puberty. Until the child's face has grown, medications and appliances may be needed to correct the obstructive sleep apnea.

Tracheostomy: Since the obstruction occurs in most children at the level of the back of the tongue, bypassing this area will resolve the problem. A tracheostomy is a tube that is placed into the windpipe (the trachea) through a small hole that is made just above the breastbone, at the bottom of the neck. The child is then able to breathe through this small hole, bypassing the obstruction. If the obstruction only occurs during sleep, then the tracheostomy can be 'plugged' up during the day, allowing the child to talk and breathe normally while awake, and unplugged only during sleep, correcting the obstructive sleep apnea. Obviously, a surgical operation is required to insert the tracheostomy. This procedure is limited to the most severe cases, where there is no other treatment available.

Other surgical approaches: Other types of surgery have been tried, primarily aimed at either shrinking the soft palate (the soft parts at the back of the roof of the mouth) or reducing the size of the tongue. These major surgeries have not been very effective in children.

STEP 5: Use a Nasal CPAP Appliance

Continuous positive airway pressure (CPAP) can be applied by wearing a mask connected to a machine that delivers air through the nose and is called nasal-CPAP or n-CPAP. The airway collapses during breathing because of the negative pressure that is created during inspiration. Abolishing this negative pressure by blowing air into the nose, thereby keeping a positive pressure within the airway, will prevent this collapse from occurring. This can be accomplished by placing an airtight mask over the child's nose and blowing in air under pressure from a pump. Unfortunately, it is somewhat uncomfortable to wear an airtight mask and have air blown up your nose. Only children with the most severe sleep apnea, producing the greatest sleep fragmentation and sleepiness, should sleep with n-CPAP in place.

case study: **Kevin** (continued)

We set out to help Anne determine if Kevin simply has primary snoring or has OSAS and needs further evaluation.

Kevin is in the typical age range for developing obstructive sleep apnea syndrome. It sounds like he began to have symptoms around the age of 3 years. In the sleep diary we asked her to keep for Kevin, Anne noted that the time of the pauses in breathing was between 15 and 20 seconds. He also seemed to be suffering from sleep disruption caused by the breathing difficulties because he was showing signs of inattention and behavior problems during the day, especially in the afternoon.

We discussed with Anne other possible causes of problems at day care (such as the environment, staff, or children) to make sure that the problems could be attributed to his disturbed sleep, but there did not seem to be any significant problems in those areas. Because Anne does not smoke and does not allow others to smoke in the house, this was not a problem contributing to Kevin's possible OSA. When Kevin was examined in the clinic, his tonsils were slightly enlarged, but Anne was reminded that the size of a child's tonsils does not always tell you that this is the cause of obstruction.

We referred Kevin to an ear, nose, and throat specialist, who based on the case history and medical evaluations, determined that Kevin should have his tonsils and adenoids surgically removed. Within a few weeks of the operation, Anne was happy to relay that Kevin was no longer snoring or having pauses in his breathing. He also seemed to be getting along better at day care. Anne was able to put Kevin back in his own bedroom – and at last, she could sleep through the night.

What Is Hypoventilation?

When you breathe in, oxygen in the air is absorbed by the lungs, where it enters the bloodstream, and the waste gas (carbon dioxide) is breathed out. Hypoventilation occurs when your child is breathing, but is unable to take in enough air over time to keep the blood levels of oxygen and carbon dioxide normal. If your child is taking either too small or too few breaths, the blood gases become abnormal, resulting in low oxygen and high carbon dioxide levels.

Breath Control

While awake, breathing is controlled by a variety of different parts of the brain, including the frontal lobes, but during sleep, breathing is controlled by a single small area, called the respiratory nuclei, situated at the base of the brain.

Children with damage to the respiratory nuclei may breathe fine while awake, but once they go to sleep and the frontal lobes of the brain are no longer stimulating breathing, they lose the drive to breathe, resulting in central apnea or hypoventilation.

Causes of Hypoventilation

The muscles used in breathing may be too weak to take a big enough breath. This can occur as a result of a disease that causes muscles in general not to work well (such as muscular dystrophy) or diseases damaging the nerves that control muscles (such as polio).

Alternatively, there may be nothing wrong with the muscles themselves, but they are not strong enough for the work asked of them. This can occur if the child is excessively overweight, the weight of the tummy being too much for the major muscle of breathing, the diaphragm, to bear, or because the child's lungs are severely scarred by disease.

SYMPTOMS OF HYPOVENTILATION

To determine if your child is experiencing hypoventilation, look for these symptoms:

- Shortness of breath: Children who have disease affecting either the muscles or nerves controlling breathing are usually well aware that they have trouble breathing because they experience shortness of breath.

- Poor or disturbed sleep: During sleep, the breathing of children with hypoventilation becomes shallower, resulting in a drop in their blood oxygen level and a rise in the carbon dioxide. Since their brain stem works fine, the low oxygen and high carbon dioxide wakes them up and disturbs their sleep.

- Respiratory center damage: Children with damage to the respiratory centers may not be aware of any problems because these centers tell them there is trouble with their breathing, and, consequently, they may have remarkably few, if any, symptoms. Fortunately, the respiratory center is very well protected at the base of the skull and is rarely damaged without other, obvious evidence of brain damage.

Guidelines for Treating Hypoventilation

THE BEST TREATMENT for hypoventilation is to treat the underlying cause. However, the underlying cause is not always easily treatable.

STEP 1: Reduce Weight

If overweight or obesity is the problem, your child needs to decrease his caloric intake and burn off more calories by becoming more active. Consult with your health-care provider about strategies for helping your child with weight loss.

STEP 2: Treat the Medical Disorder

If the problem is a medical disorder and not related to obesity, discuss with your doctor ways to improve air exchange. If your doctor does not have a treatment for the cause of the hypoventilation, the best solution may be some form of ventilator that will do at least some, if not all, of the breathing for your child.

Chapter 10

Bed-Wetting (Enuresis)

I F YOUR CHILD WETS his bed, you're likely frustrated with his behavior and maybe even a bit angry at the burden of extra laundry added to your already busy schedule. You may think your child is bed-wetting because he is too lazy to get out of bed or he is doing this out of anger or unhappiness with you. None of these reasons is true, however. Children who bed-wet do so in deep sleep and are completely unaware of the need to urinate at the time of the bed-wetting episode. If your child bed-wets, he is not bad, angry, depressed, or lazy. He's just sleeping.

Still, your child's sleep may be affected by his bed-wetting because he will be disturbed when he becomes uncomfortable from the dampness and wakens at night. Although he may be able to change his pajamas and linen quickly or place a dry towel on the bed and get back to sleep easily without having significant sleep disruption, bed-wetting can affect your child's self-esteem, relationships with his friends, and his relationship with you, his parents.

What Is Nocturnal Enuresis (Bed-Wetting)?

Enuresis means incontinence of urine in children who should have outgrown it. When your child has enuresis, he may experience this problem while awake (diurnal) or while sleeping (nocturnal). The two types of enuresis (diurnal and nocturnal) are very different conditions with different causes and treatments. This chapter deals with primary nocturnal enuresis, commonly called bed-wetting. If your child has secondary enuresis or diurnal enuresis you should discuss these problems with your health-care provider.

There are effective treatments available for older children and teenagers who are bothered by bed-wetting.

Did You Know?

Prevalence and Prognosis
Bed-wetting is found in 10% to 15% of 5-year-olds and 6% to 8% of 8-year-olds, declining to 1% to 2% of the population by age 15. Bed-wetting is slightly more common in boys. Younger children who have primary nocturnal enuresis (which means that they have not slept dry for 6 consecutive months) and only wet at night will usually outgrow the problem over time.

Bed-Wetting Definition
- The child wets the bed regularly (more than twice weekly).
- The child is more than 5 years old.
- The child has never had 6 dry months in a row.

TYPES OF ENURESIS

Diurnal enuresis: A child experiencing diurnal enuresis may wet his pants during the day when awake, and he may also wet the bed at night when sleeping.

Nocturnal enuresis: A child experiencing nocturnal enuresis wets the bed only during sleep, usually deep sleep.

Each type of enuresis can also be divided by whether or not your child has ever stopped wetting or been toilet trained.

Primary enuresis: If your child has primary enuresis, he has always wet and has never been toilet trained for a significant period of time.

Secondary enuresis: If your child stopped wetting for at least 6 months and then restarted, he has secondary enuresis.

Causes of Bed-Wetting

Deep Sleep

One of the factors contributing to bed-wetting is deep sleep. Studies have shown that bed-wetting children are more difficult to wake up during the night and have brain-wave patterns demonstrating deeper sleep. While diurnal (daytime) accidents and secondary enuresis may be caused by a number of issues, primary enuresis (bed-wetting) is not due to any medical or psychological problem — these kids simply don't wake up when they have to urinate.

Genetics

Enuresis is inherited. Usually, but not always, one of the parents of a child with enuresis is a deeper sleeper and will often find out that they also wet the bed when they go back and ask their own parents. Normal sleep patterns change as children develop. Your child will naturally have less deep sleep as he gets older. That is why most children who wet their bed will outgrow this problem. Fifteen percent of children with enuresis will outgrow it each year. Your child may be showing signs of outgrowing it simply by having more and more dry nights between wet nights.

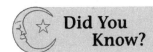
Did You Know?

Primary Nocturnal Enuresis

The most common type of enuresis is primary nocturnal enuresis, which means your child only wets the bed during sleep, is dry during the day when awake, and has had no significant period of time (less than 6 months) of being dry consistently at night.

case study: **Ethan**

When Ethan came to our clinic, he was 11 years old and wet the bed once or twice a week. His parents worried that he had a bladder problem or a behavior problem because his younger sister is already dry at night. They have tried waking him up at midnight to get him to urinate (which he does, half-asleep), but then wets the bed a few hours later. He wakes up at about 5:00 a.m. when his sheets get cold and asks his mom to change them. His parents are at their wits' end.

Ethan is healthy and appears happy, but his parents continue to wonder if something is troubling him. He is (nearly) a straight-A student, who makes friends easily. His friends want him to come to camp with him this summer, but he is afraid to go and be 'found-out'. Ethan and his parents are not sure what to do. They don't want him to go to camp and be teased by other children....

(continued page 198)

Guidelines for Treating Bed-Wetting

NO BEHAVIORAL OR medical treatment is necessary for primary nocturnal enuresis. Remember, nocturnal enuresis is not voluntary; it is due to deep sleep and resolves with time. If you choose to start a treatment for enuresis for your child when he isn't bothered by the bed-wetting, the treatment might make your child believe that she is doing something very wrong that needs to stop. Help your child understand that there is nothing wrong and that bed-wetting is simply a problem that results from deep sleep.

However, older children and teenagers may not want to wait to outgrow it. In certain situations, such as when your child wants to sleep at a friend or relative's home, treatment may be desirable. If the enuresis is really troubling your child, there are several treatment options.

STEP 1: Use Alarm Devices

Enuresis alarms are connected to a pad placed on the bed that is sensitive to small amounts of liquid. These alarms are used to teach children to wake to the sensation of a full bladder by associating a loud noise with the first few drops of urine that touch the pad.

For teenagers who are fed up with their bed-wetting and motivated to try another solution, the alarm option offers better results than other treatment options in terms of staying dry once the treatment stops. Research studies tell us that the alarms 'cure' enuresis in about half of the children who try it. Other treatments may be less trouble and work just fine during treatment, but are temporary measures only.

Families must be very motivated to use these devices because they need to be used consistently every night for several months. The alarms often wake up other sleepers in the house. It is also difficult to use the alarm when your child is sleeping out, at summer camp or at a friend's house, for example. They are also expensive.

STEP 2: Use Medications

Several medications are commonly prescribed for bed-wetting, with modest results.

Desmopressin: Desmopressin (DDAVP) is a form of antidiuretic hormone produced in our bodies. The medication can be administered as a pill or nasal spray to be taken 1 hour before bedtime. DDAVP signals the kidneys to reduce the amount of urine produced, then makes up for the amount during the day. Desmopressin is probably best suited for use in preventing bed-wetting at sleepovers. It is not recommended for long-term use in the treatment of nocturnal enuresis.

Imipramine: Imipramine is a pill taken at night that probably works by altering sleep patterns. Imipramine, in small doses, generally works safely and about as well as desmopressin. Like desmopressin, it works for most, but not all, children with enuresis on the nights the medication is taken, but not after the medication is stopped. If an accidental overdose occurs, imipramine is much more dangerous than desmopressin and may even be fatal. You need to ensure that it is stored safely out of reach of your children. For this reason, imipramine is now seldom recommended unless other treatments have been tried without success, and then only with caution.

EVALUATE BEHAVIORAL THERAPIES

A recent summary of studies published on behavioral therapies for enuresis concluded that it was not clear whether or not more good or more harm was being done by behavioral therapies for enuresis. You will need to evaluate these treatments with your health-care provider before proceding.

Rewards and Punishments: Health-care providers in the past have commonly recommended behavior modification strategies, such as rewards for dry nights. It is difficult to convince a child that a wet night is nothing to be ashamed of when we reward dry nights. The failure to win the reward may further diminish a child's self-esteem. Punishments and rewards for an involuntary action should both be avoided. Wetting the bed while sleeping is not a choice children make.

Waking Your Child: Waking your child to go in the toilet ('lifting') to empty the bladder is often difficult for both parent and child and usually doesn't work.

Bladder Training: Training your child to hold his urine as long as possible during the day is also difficult and also not very effective.

No Link to Emotional Problems: Parents often worry that their child's bed-wetting must be due, in part, to an emotional problem because they wet the bed in one setting but not in another. For example, some children wet the bed while sleeping at home, but not at their grandparent's home. Children often do have wet nights in one home, but not their other home. This is likely due to different depths of sleep in different settings, not an emotional problem.

Tips for Treating Bed-Wetting

1. **Reduce the amount of fluids just before bedtime:** Do not limit fluids at dinnertime. Have your child empty his bladder at bedtime.

2. **Use protective bedding:** Be sure that you and your child are not anxious or concerned with damaging the mattress from the bed-wetting.

3. **Consider training pants:** Training pants that do not look like diapers can be used. Only use these if your child does not feel self-conscious. If you believe that your child is wetting while lying awake in bed, then you should try a few nights without them.

4. **Decrease skin irritation from damp clothes:** Avoid tight underwear and use barrier creams (such as petroleum jelly) so that when your child does wet, his skin will be less likely to become irritated.

5. **Make sure that your child has no barriers to get to the toilet at night:** For example, fear of the dark can be helped by keeping a night-light on in the bathroom.

6. **If you include your child in morning cleanup of the soiled bedclothes and bed sheets, do this in a positive, non-punitive manner:** Try saying, for example, "You're a big boy now so you can help the grown-ups."

7. **Avoid showing your frustration:** Remember, your child is bed-wetting while he is in a deep sleep. This is involuntary.

Q. When should we worry about bed-wetting?

A. Almost all children will outgrow enuresis eventually. If they are not ashamed of their bed-wetting, if they understand that it is not their fault that it is neither an emotional nor medical problem, they are not likely to suffer any psychological damage from bed-wetting as an older child or teenager.

However, you should visit your health-care provider if your child is wetting for these reasons:

- If your child begins to wet the bed again after having been dry at night for at least 6 months (this is called secondary enuresis)

- If your child begins to wet himself during the day when awake (this is called diurnal enuresis)

- If your child develops excessive thirst and awakens in the night by thirst, loses weight and energy, experiences blurred vision or a significant change in appetite

- If your child develops back pain, stomach pain, or a burning sensation when he urinates

- If your child begins to have smaller, more frequent daytime urination or if he always has to rush to the bathroom to make it on time

- If your child begins to have difficulty not only with bladder control, but also with bowel control – that is, if soiling with stool occurs

- If your child develops any weakness in the legs or if there are sudden changes in your child's gait (how legs look when walking)

- If your child appears to have any fainting spells, convulsions, or subtle, unusual movements before wetting

- If your child is excessively sleepy during the daytime

- If your child has an unusual birthmark or tuft of hair on the lower back, in the middle, just above his buttocks, which could be a sign of a problem in the spinal cord

case study: **Ethan** (continued)

We agreed with Ethan and his parents that he should not miss going to camp because of his bed-wetting anxiety. For the short term, we prescribed desmopressin (DDAVP) in a pill or nasal spray, to be taken each night 1 hour before bed for the 2 weeks he will be away at summer camp. We explained that the medication reduces the amount of urine made for the night so that the bladder does not fill up.

Ethan decided to try the nasal for a week before making his final decision about attending camp. He was happy to find that it works. If he is still wetting the bed when it comes time to go to camp, he can use the DDAVP and remain dry at night.

Ethan signed up for camp in the winter, but by the spring he no longer wet the bed or needs medication.

Chapter 11

Restless Legs Syndrome (RLS)

WHEN YOUR CHILD climbs into bed with you to sleep, do you feel her periodically kicking you during the night? Some children are more restless than others while sleeping. However, all restlessness is not a problem. You should be worried if this restlessness is associated with another sleep problem, such as snoring or bed-wetting. You should also be concerned if your restless child has trouble falling asleep due to funny sensations in his legs at night, or in addition to his restlessness appears to be getting adequate sleep but has symptoms of daytime sleepiness, irritability, and/or poor attention. Then your child may be suffering from restless legs syndrome or an associated condition, periodic limb movement disorder (PLMD).

Restless legs syndrome and periodic limb movement disorder often occur together. While RLS and PLMD have been studied extensively in adults, sleep experts have just started to evaluate these problems in children. We do know that RLS and PLMD can disrupt sleep and that sleep disruption can lead to daytime problems with attention. The information in this chapter is largely based on research in adults with restless legs syndrome.

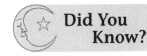

Did You Know?

Prevalence of Restless Legs Syndrome
The prevalence of RLS is between 5% and 15% in adults. It is primarily a problem of middle-age adults, and the older you get, the more common the problem. We do not know how often it is seen in children.

What Is Restless Legs Syndrome?

Restless legs syndrome (RLS) is a sleep disorder that is well recognized in adults. This syndrome is characterized by the irresistible urge to move the limbs, predominantly in the evening or at night. This is usually accompanied by a peculiar discomfort, pain, or burning feeling in the lower extremities, which may be described as a "creepy" or "crawly" feeling. The result of having this problem in the evening is difficulty falling asleep and staying asleep, which can lead to daytime symptoms of fatigue and inattention. Usually, the desire is to move the legs, but it can also include an uncomfortable feeling and the urge to move the arms.

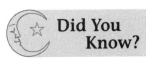

Did You Know?

PLMD and RLS
Not all people with restless legs syndrome have periodic limb movement disorder (PLMD). In adults with RLS, the majority (about 85%) will have PLMD. You can have RLS, but not PLMD. We don't know how often children with RLS will also have PLMD.

Periodic Limb Movement Disorder

Periodic limb movement disorder (PLMD) occurs in about 85% of people with RLS during sleep. PLMD usually occurs during sleep and less often during wakefulness. In RLS, the urge to move and the actual movement of your legs is voluntary. In PMLD, these movements are involuntary, not under your control, and periodic. PMLD is diagnosed only with a formal sleep study of the frequency and strength of the movements.

PLMD Diagnosis

Whether PLMD is a significant problem will be determined by assessing other symptoms your child has during the day or during sleep and the results of an overnight sleep laboratory test, which is used to evaluate the actual number and frequency of leg kicking during the night.

In PLMD, you have repetitive episodes of at least four movements of your legs, which last from 0.5 to 5 seconds and recur at intervals from 20 to 40 seconds. It is considered a problem if you have more than five episodes of this type of movement per hour of sleep on average. The movement may cause a partial arousal from sleep, but you are usually not aware of being awake at night because it is brief. However, this involuntary movement during sleep can disrupt your sleep, leading to daytime symptoms from disturbed sleep.

Symptoms of Restless Legs Syndrome

With RLS, your child will feel forced to move around to get relief from these symptoms, by turning in bed, pacing, shaking, rubbing his legs, or getting up and walking around. These symptoms are present or get worse when he rests, but when he moves around, there is a partial and temporary relief. At the beginning, when this disorder develops, it is not a constant problem, but with time, it can become a continuous and chronic problem.

Symptoms of RLS

The following criteria for diagnosing RLS in adults and children have been established by an international group of experts on this condition, published in the journal *Sleep Medicine* (2003).

Did You Know?

Restless Rhythms
Symptoms of restless legs syndrome are worse in the evening or night. Whether you are sleeping or not, the symptoms will be worse between midnight and 4:00 a.m., and be the least bothersome between 6:00 and 10:00 am. Sleep is disturbed in 95% of people with this disorder, resulting in daytime symptoms of inadequate sleep.

Four symptoms are essential for the diagnosis of RLS in adults:

- An urge to move the legs is usually accompanied by uncomfortable or unpleasant sensations in the legs.

- Unpleasant sensations or the urge to move will begin or get worse during periods of rest of inactivity, such as lying or sitting.

- Unpleasant sensations or the urge to move are partly or totally relieved by movement, such as walking, bending, or stretching, for at least as long as the activity continues.

- Unpleasant sensations or the urge to move are worse in the evening or at night than during the day, or only occur in the evening or night.

Three other features of RLS may be present to support the diagnosis in adults but are not essential:

- Adults will have a good response to treatment with drugs that increase the level of dopamine in the brain

- Movements of the limbs at specific intervals while awake or sleeping

- Family history of RLS

To confirm diagnosis of RLS in children, they must present the following symptoms:

- All four adult symptoms, plus the child must relate a description in his own words that is consistent with leg discomfort

OR

- All four adult symptoms, plus two or three of the following symptoms:

- Sleep disturbance for age

- Biologic parent or sibling with a definite diagnosis of RLS

- Sleep study showing there are periodic limb movements during sleep at a minimum frequency. The sleep experts define this as at least five or more movements an hour.

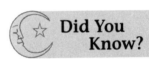

Did You Know?

Early Onset

A large survey by the American Restless Legs Foundation determined that approximately 45% of people with RLS report their symptoms starting before the age of 20 years.

QUESTIONNAIRE FOR DIAGNOSING RLS IN CHILDREN

You can determine if your child has restless legs syndrome by answering the following questions. It is suggested that you do not ask your child these questions directly; rather, observe your child and listen to his description of his restlessness. If you ask your child if he has "creepy" feelings in his legs, it is possible that this will suggest the feeling to him. Check off "Yes" answers and cross out "No" answers with an 'X' in the boxes.

1. Sensations and Activities

❏ Does your child describe an urge to move or use words to describe an unpleasant sensation in his legs?

❏ Do you observe or does your child describe these feelings during times when he is resting?

❏ Do you observe or does your child describe these feelings more in the evening and at night than in the daytime?

❏ Does your child prefer to walk, rock, or do other activities at night to relieve this feeling in his legs?

❏ Does your child tell you that this activity helps him to decrease the unpleasant sensations in his legs?

❏ Does your child have trouble sitting at a movie or while on a bus, car, or airplane because of these feelings?

2. Sleep Disturbance

❏ Does your child have difficulty falling asleep at night?

❏ Does your child relate this problem of falling asleep to, or do you observe it to be related to, these feelings in his legs?

❏ Does your child wake frequently at night?

❏ Does your child get adequate sleep at night, but not appear to be well rested?

❏ Does your child appear more restless than you would expect at night, especially with kicking of the legs?

3. Family History

❏ Do you or your partner or other close family members have a diagnosis of RLS?

If you answered "Yes" to many of the questions in Part 1, or "Yes" to some of the questions in Part 1 but also to the questions in Part 2 and 3, you should review these concerns with your child's health-care provider.

Causes of Restless Legs Syndrome

There are two main causes of RLS — genetic factors (which means that your child inherited the disease) and symptomatic causes (which means your child acquired the disease in association with another medical problem or as a side effect of taking medications).

Genetic Factors

There is probably a genetic cause to RLS because in adults who do not have a cause for their RLS, the majority have a positive family history (63% to 92%). There are some large families where it has occurred in enough family members to study the genetic basis, but the exact way that the disease is inherited is still not known. The inheritance of this problem is complex and not known to be caused by a single genetic defect.

However, there is evidence for an inherited form in children with possible RLS who have a family member with the same problem. Even when it appears to be related to genetics, there are probably other factors that influence who will develop symptoms in the family.

Symptomatic Causes

RLS may be caused by other specific medical problems:
- Iron deficiency (the most frequent cause)
- Pregnancy (also may be related to having low iron stores)
- Severe kidney disease
- Diabetes
- Rheumatoid arthritis

Drugs

Some foods and drugs have been reported to cause RLS, or if you have RLS, make the symptoms worse:
- Caffeine
- Sedating antihistamines
- Some drugs used for stomach problems to avoid vomiting, such as metoclopramide
- Calcium channel blockers
- Some antidepressants (tricyclic antidepressants) and selective serotonin reuptake inhibitors, or SSRIs. SSRIs may worsen or relieve symptoms of RLS.

Restless Legs Sensations
Here are some of the ways that children may describe the feelings in their legs with RLS:
- Creepy-crawly
- Ouchies
- Bugs or ants crawling inside legs or on legs
- Throbbing
- Tingling
- Burning
- Want to move legs, or energy in legs
- Tickling

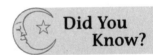 **Did You Know?**

RLS and Iron Deficiency
Iron is necessary for the production of dopamine in the brain. The concentration of iron in the body has a circadian rhythm — there is a drop in concentration of iron at night, which is the time when the symptoms of RLS become worse. Drugs that produce more dopamine are used to treat RLS.

Other Causes of Restlessness and Leg Kicking at Night

Other sleep disorders may be confused with RLS. Your child may be restless because she is anxious or cannot fall asleep. Many people have jerks as they fall asleep called sleep myoclonus. This

case study: Pierre

Antoinette and Frederique brought their 13-year-old son, Pierre, to our clinic concerned about his behavior, both at school and at home. Pierre is a bright boy, who has been in a special class for gifted students since Grade 3. However, his teacher has been concerned over the last year because Pierre is not paying attention, fidgets during class, and is easily distracted. She has asked Antoinette to have a health-care practitioner see if Pierre has attention deficit/hyperactivity disorder (ADHD).

When we asked the family about Pierre's sleep, this is what they described. There are five children (all boys) in the home, ranging from 2 years to 16 years of age. Frederique works a night shift and leaves the home at 7:00 p.m., returning in the morning just before the children go to school. The home is somewhat chaotic in the evening, with Antoinette trying to attend to all the children's needs. She is able to get the two youngest boys (ages 2 and 5 years) to bed at a reasonable time, but admits that she has no control over Pierre and his older brothers.

Pierre goes to sleep when he wants (sometimes as late as midnight), and on the weekend, his schedule is very erratic. When he does go to bed, it takes him 45 to 60 minutes to fall asleep. We discussed other issues related to sleep hygiene and it appears that Pierre (and his brothers) enjoy energy drinks especially in the evening. Antoinette had no idea about the amount of caffeine in these drinks.

Pierre added, without prompting, that he feels funny sensations in his legs, which he says are worse when he is watching television or playing on his computer (which are both in his bedroom) and when he is tired in the evening. We asked him to describe these feelings, and he said "like a shock of lightening" and "sometimes like a spider crawling up my veins." He says that he can make the feelings go away by rubbing his legs or walking around, but they seem to always return.

His parents think that maybe Pierre is making up these sensations because he may not feel he is getting enough attention. Antoinette has never told Pierre that she has restless legs syndrome, so as not to worry him, but she recognizes the symptoms that he is describing and thinks he may have the same problem. The family also wants to know if Pierre should be tested for ADHD....

(continued on page 207)

is a normal way that the body moves from the waking to the sleep state. Muscle cramps tend to get worse at night, as do panic attacks. Seizures may also cause leg movements at night. Periodic leg movements can occur in other sleep disorders or diseases of the nervous system. Periodic limb movement disorder can also cause similar symptoms to RLS.

Possibility of RLS in Children Who Are Inattentive

While RLS and PLMD have been studied extensively in adults, sleep experts have just started to evaluate these problems in children. We know that RLS and/or PLMD, when it occurs in children, can disrupt their sleep, as it does in adults, and lead to daytime problems with attention. It is possible that some children who are diagnosed with attention deficit/hyperactivity disorder (ADHD) have problems with sleep, such as RLS or PLMD, causing their inattentive symptoms, but we do not know how commonly this occurs. These children may not respond to conventional behavioral or pharmacologic management of ADHD. If you think that your child has symptoms of RLS or another sleep disorder, you should review this with your health-care provider.

Guidelines for Treating Restless Legs Syndrome

THE TREATMENT FOR restless legs syndrome in adults is well known (including improving sleep hygiene, providing iron supplementation if iron levels are low, and using specific drugs), but the treatment in children has not been well researched because the diagnosis is not made frequently. Even in adults with definite diagnosis of RLS, not everyone needs to be treated with medication. It depends on the severity of the symptoms and if other measures to improve sleep hygiene are sufficient.

If you think that your child has restless legs syndrome, there are some treatments that can be helpful in decreasing motor restlessness. If these strategies do not help, then you should consult with your health-care provider.

STEP 1: Educate Yourself and Your Child

Parents and children need to learn about the problem as part of the treatment plan. You can educate yourself by reading this book and other sleep books, by reviewing the RLS Internet sites (see the "Resources" section in this book), and by asking your health-care provider questions about your child's condition.

STEP 2: Improve Sleep Hygiene

If your child's sleep is disrupted by any sleep disorder, it is always going to help to have a regular schedule, to promote adequate and continuous sleep, and to decrease the impact of sleep problems on daytime function. For more guidelines in establishing proper sleep hygiene, see Part 1, Chapter 3, "Sleep Hygiene."

STEP 3: Exercise and Employ Relaxation Strategies

In adults, it is known that moderate exercise before bed may suppress symptoms, but either vigorous exercise or being immobile for a long time may make the symptoms worse. Simple relaxation strategies, such as massage and a warm bath in the evening, may also be helpful.

STEP 4: Avoid Problematic Foods and Drugs

Any substance that interferes with normal sleep will exacerbate the symptoms of RLS. Be sure your child avoids caffeinated foods, beverages, and drugs for at least 6 hours before bedtime. If this does not improve his symptoms, try to eliminate all caffeine from your child's diet.

STEP 5: Be Mentally Active

If you can get your child's mind off of the symptoms of restlessness in the evening, this may be helpful. Try activities that require concentration, such as crossword puzzles, soduko, and nonviolent video games, for example.

STEP 6: Check Iron Stores

If your child is diagnosed with RLS or PLMD, his health-care provider may check the iron levels in his blood and recommend taking iron supplements if needed.

STEP 7: Use Medications

Several types of drugs can be helpful in adults with RLS of PMD, including benzodiazepines, some anti-seizure medications, and drugs that increase the level of dopamine. Opioids (which are narcotics), such as codeine, can be used in adults with caution due to their significant side effects. Not all people with RLS or PLMD require medications. Your health-care provider will discuss the use of medications if a diagnosis is confirmed in your child.

Q. When should I consult a doctor about my child's restless leg behavior?

A. Contact your doctor if your child has most of the symptoms described in this chapter and listed in the questionnaire, plus one or more of the following – a family member with RLS; sleep disturbance or difficulty with falling asleep and waking frequently at night; or daytime difficulties with memory, mood, behavior, attention, or learning.

Q. What is the relationship between 'growing pains' and RLS?

A. 'Growing pains' are a common problem among children. Between 3% and 34% have been reported to experience these pains in six research studies of this problem. The children experience muscular aches in the legs that occur late in the day or during the night that may waken children from sleep. At this time, we do not have enough research to know if there are some children with 'growing pains' who also have symptoms of RLS or will go on to develop RLS.

case study: **Pierre** (continued)

Based on the history provided by Pierre and his family, we made the diagnosis of restless legs syndrome. In addition to his symptoms, Antoinette has RLS, which makes it likely that he has a genetic cause.

Pierre's poor sleep hygiene and excessive caffeine use also contribute to his sleep problems, which have resulted in inattention, hyperactivity, and distractibility at school. These problems may be a result of the sleep disruption from his RLS or he may have both RLS and ADHD. We decided to investigate further. Pierre's iron level was found to be normal. He was referred for an overnight sleep study, which showed that he had trouble falling asleep in the laboratory, but he did not have periodic limb movement disorder (PLMD). Pierre was asked to cut out all caffeine, and his parents were advised to improve the sleep hygiene for all their children.

We saw Pierre in our clinic 3 months later. He brought a 2-week sleep diary to this follow-up visit. He was very proud to show us that his sleep schedule was much more regular. Since making the changes in his sleep schedule, he is reportedly concentrating better at school.

Chapter 12

Teeth Grinding and Gnashing (Bruxism)

THERE ARE MANY NOISES that can be irritating to hear, the sound of a child or adult grinding and gnashing their teeth being high on the list. Once you hear this grating, crunching sound, technically called bruxism, you will never forget it.

What do you do if you hear this sound coming from your child's room while he is sleeping? Consider your options: buy earplugs, insulate the bedroom door, or try to ignore the sound (the hardest option) and get some sleep? Although the sound of your child grinding his teeth can be grating on your nerves (pardon the pun), in general, this sleep disturbance may disrupt your sleep, but will not affect your child's sleep and may not have any adverse effect on his teeth.

What Is Bruxism?

Bruxism is repetitive gnashing and grinding of teeth associated with clenching of the jaws. Children can grind their teeth when awake or asleep. This is involuntary — and normal, unless done excessively. The teeth grinding and gnashing may or may not cause noise. Children who have neurological problems, such as developmental delay or cerebral palsy, are at risk for developing bruxism; however, it can also be seen in healthy children. In healthy children, bruxism is not usually associated with any significant consequences.

Bruxism tends to occur in children during two periods of their development — when the baby teeth erupt in infants and toddlers and between 5 and 10 years of age, when the permanent teeth erupt until all the teeth are present. There are few consequences of bruxism in children because the baby teeth do not stay in place long enough for any permanent damage and because bruxism usually stops in childhood before any permanent damage can occur to the adult teeth. Studies in adults show that about 8% of adults report bruxism and about 4% (or one-half of those who report it) have consequences from teeth grinding.

Did You Know?

Prevalence of Bruxism
While there are only a few studies on the frequency of bruxism in children, bruxism is reported to occur in 14% to 20% of children. Approximately 50% of children who are reported to have bruxism stop by 10 years of age.

SYMPTOMS OF PROBLEMATIC BRUXISM

Bruxism in your child may be a problem if one or more of the following symptoms are present:

- If you hear a grinding or grating sound of bruxism while your child is sleeping that is loud enough to disturb you or other family members
- If your dentist notices excessive destruction of your child's teeth or early loss of teeth
- If your child complains of sensitive teeth (if, for example, hot or cold foods or liquids cause tooth pain)
- If your child complains when he wakes in the morning of a headache, earache, toothache, pain in the facial muscles or in the jaw joint

ASSOCIATED SYMPTOMS

Bruxism can be associated with symptoms of other sleep-related and medical conditions:

- Upper airway obstruction from enlarged tonsils and/or adenoids
- Other sleep disturbances, such as bed-wetting, sleep talking
- One study showed that children were more likely to have bruxism if someone else in the family had bruxism, slept with open bedroom doors, were mouth breathers or drooled, or were reported to have psychological disorders.

Causes of Bruxism

Factors Increasing Bruxism

It is not entirely clear what causes bruxism, but several factors may increase it:

- Response to pain, such as with a cold or earache, or teething. The child may grind teeth to ease the pain, like you would rub a sore muscle. Grinding may also help to relieve pressure in the eustachian tube, which connects the inner ear to the inside of the throat.
- Allergies. Teeth grinding may relieve the itching, sneezing, and coughing associated with allergies.
- Stress and anxiety. The mechanism of this association between stress, anxiety, and bruxism are unclear, but it is known that reducing stress and anxiety can be effective in decreasing the symptoms of bruxism.

- Family history. If your child grinds his teeth, it's likely one of your close family members also grinds his or her teeth.

- In the past, it was thought that an abnormal bite and crooked or missing teeth could contribute to the development of bruxism, but recently this is felt to be less important. If your child has these problems, discuss their relevance to his teeth grinding with your dentist.

Factors Associated with Bruxism

Studies have shown that certain factors are associated with bruxism in adults, but there is not enough research in children to know if this also applies to them. These factors may be significant in teenagers who have significant bruxism:

- Moderate daytime sleepiness

- Use of alcohol, caffeine, and nicotine

case study: Mohammed

Mohammed is a 9-year-old boy who is small for his age, and has always been shy and self-conscious of his size. In the past, he was always happy to go to school with a small group of friends who have been together since kindergarten. His parents brought him to our sleep clinic because, since moving to a new neighborhood, they have been hearing disturbing sounds of teeth grinding at night when Mohammed is sleeping. The problem began 6 months ago when the family moved from the north to the south end of the city. Mohammed started going to a new school after the winter break in the middle of the school year. Mohammed's parents knew that he was nervous about this change, but they had no choice because Mohammed's father was changing jobs.

The clenching and grinding of teeth are heard about twice a week and the noise is loud enough to disturb both parents' sleep. His parents are not sure if Mohammed was grinding his teeth before they moved or if this is a new habit that he has developed. They are now hearing the sounds because they live in a smaller house with their bedrooms closer together. His parents know that Mohammed is not happy at school and is having trouble making friends, but they did not realize that this stress might be related to Mohammed's teeth grinding. His parents want to know what to do – should they ignore the sound or be concerned about Mohammed's dental or general health?....

(continued on page 212)

Guidelines for Treating Bruxism

STEP 1: Consult with Your Dentist

If your child grinds or gnashes her teeth while sleeping, talk to your dentist. He can evaluate if there is damage to your child's teeth. If there is tooth wear, your dentist may simply need to examine your child more frequently or suggest a dental appliance for your child to wear at night to protect the teeth.

STEP 2: Consult with Your Health-Care Provider

Talk to your health-care provider if you have any concerns about your child's teeth grinding — for example, if your child wakes in the morning with headaches, earaches, or facial pain. Also talk to your doctor about possible causes of stress, the most likely factor contributing to your child's bruxism, and how to reduce stress.

STEP 3: Reduce Stress

Decreasing stress is suggested for adults who have sleep bruxism, but it is not known if this is helpful in children. Adults can decrease stress by increasing their relaxing evening activities, such as reading a book or taking a warm bath. You can try similar techniques with your child to help him develop relaxing bedtime routines at night. Older children and adults can also use relaxation or other techniques to decrease stress. It is also helpful to reduce stress for your child by finding the cause, although it may be more complicated and require further psychological evaluation.

STEP 4: Relieve Pain

If your child has significant jaw pain from the grinding, applying a warm wet washcloth to the side of the face may help relax the muscles.

STEP 5: Use Medications

There are medications used in adults for sleep bruxism, though drugs have not been studied and would rarely be prescribed for children to treat bruxism.

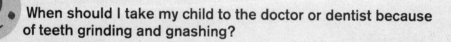

Q. When should I take my child to the doctor or dentist because of teeth grinding and gnashing?

A. You should see your dentist if you have any of the following concerns about your child's grinding, whether it is a new problem or an ongoing problem:

- If your child appears to also be anxious, stressed, or has other behavioral problems that could be related to underlying stress

- If your child complains of jaw problems, such as pain or difficulty in opening his jaw

- If your child complains of morning headaches, earaches, or facial pain

- If your child complains when eating hot or cold food due to tooth sensitivity

- If the jaw movement is very repetitive or stereotyped (which means that the movement always looks the same) and occurring with any other signs that may be part of a seizure, such as drooling, other repetitive limb movement, inability to be easily woken, self-injury, breathing difficulty, daytime fatigue or any other unusual change you observe in your child.

case study: **Mohammed** (continued)

We informed Mohammed's parents that teeth grinding during sleep is usually not a problem in childhood and should stop in time. We also advised them to talk more with Mohammed about the stress he is experiencing because of the move.

After meeting in the clinic, Mohammed's parents visited his school and spoke to his teacher. They learned that he was having difficulty fitting in, but were told there were no other problems at school with his behavior or progress. His parents spoke to Mohammed about this stress, and together they decided to invite some of the boys who lived in the neighborhood to their home after school. During the next few months, Mohammed made friends and seemed happier with his new school.

His parents ignored the noises at night from his teeth grinding, closing their door so that they could sleep. To be sure he was not damaging his teeth, they took Mohammed to their dentist.

We made a plan to monitor Mohammed's sleep bruxism, and if it did not stop at the end of 6 months, we would refer him to a counselor to be evaluated further for other sources of stress. But 6 months later, the bruxism had stopped on its own.

Chapter 13

Rhythmic Movement Disorder

WHEN YOU GO TO SLEEP at night, you may find it soothing to fall asleep in a certain way. For example, you may tuck your pillow under your chin in a particular manner, lie on your side, or even count sheep to make the transition from being awake to falling asleep. Your child may have found his own way to make this transition.

To make this transition, many children develop a soothing repetitive motion, rocking their bodies, banging their heads, or other rocking motions that help them fall asleep. These are all normal ways to fall asleep. Once asleep the movements stop. Although this type of sleep-related activity is called a rhythmic movement disorder, in most children it is not really a disorder, but a normal way that young children fall asleep. The movements are seen when your child is transitioning between sleep and wake, and when he has brief arousals from sleep during the night. In most children, no changes or treatment are needed, and with time, the rhythmic behavior just stops on its own.

What Is a Rhythmic Movement Disorder?

Rhythmic movement disorder includes a group of movements usually seen in early childhood that occurs during the transition between sleep and wake states, both at bedtime and naptimes, during arousals from sleep at night, and sometimes during light sleep. The movements are stereotyped, which means they look the same, and they are repetitive and rhythmic, as the name of the disorder suggests. When the movements occur, they usually last less than 15 minutes. The movements are more associated with sleep, but some children will do the same movements while awake.

Usually, the large muscles of the body, often in the head and neck, are involved. The movement frequently involves body-rocking and head-banging, which can be disturbing to parents.

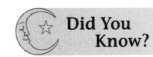

Did You Know?

Incidence of Rhythmic Movement Disorder (RMD)
RMD commonly occurs in infants and toddlers and usually resolves around the second or third year of life. About two-thirds of healthy children display some sort of RMD by 9 months of age. Children with autism, developmental delay, and other developmental disorders may develop movements at a later age or have RMD that persists to an older age. While RMD rarely persists into adulthood, it can occur even in healthy adults.

TYPES OF RHYTHMIC MOVEMENT DISORDER

- Head-banging (the most common movement) involves banging the head into the pillow, mattress, headboard, or wall while either lying down, sitting up, or rocking on hands and knees.

- Head-rolling consists of side-to-side head movements.

- Body-rocking may involve the entire body or it may be limited to the upper body with the child sitting.

- Body-rolling, leg-banging, or leg-rolling; however, they are less common.

- Rhythmic humming or chanting may accompany any of the rhythmic movements and may be quite loud.

Causes of Rhythmic Movement Disorder

While we do not know for certain what causes RMD, several factors that increase the possibility of your child developing this habit have been identified.

Did You Know?

Little Chance of Harm
Almost two-thirds of healthy children engage in this type of rhythmic movement, but there are only a few reports in the scientific literature of children causing themselves harm. The only child at risk is one who has an underlying medical, psychiatric, or developmental disorder.

Family History

Family history is important. Children who have RMD may have a close family member with the same problem.

Sleep Disruption

Anything that causes your child to wake at night will increase the opportunity for the rhythmic movement to occur. Children often have the movements when falling asleep or transitioning through the night from wake to sleep. Factors disrupting sleep include medical problems (such as a recurrent ear infection, trouble breathing at night, reflux of stomach acid causing heartburn-like symptoms) and environmental factors (noise, for example).

Attention Seeking

Your child may display this movement as a means of getting your attention at night when he is falling asleep or during arousals from sleep in the middle of the night.

Pleasure

The movement may give your child pleasure and be a form of self-stimulation, especially if your child has a neurological problem, such as autism, developmental delay, or has emotional problems.

Inner Ear Stimulation

Children may use rhythmic movements to stimulate the inner
ear, called the vestibular system. It is possible that this sensation
is soothing, but the actual explanation for this is unknown.

---

case history: **Erin**

Erin is a healthy 3-year-old who was referred to our sleep clinic because of
her unusual sleep habits. She has a regular, consistent bedtime routine.
However, since the age of 6 months, starting when she was in a crib and
continuing when she moved into a regular bed, Erin has developed a habit of
perching on her hands and knees and rocking her body in a rhythmic pattern
when falling asleep. Occasionally, her parents hear the same activity during
the night, and when they go to her, she appears to be doing this while asleep.

Her parents have tried to stop this habit without success. They have
enrolled Erin in a gym class for children, where she gets lots of chance to
move around, and they have tried putting her to bed earlier or later than
normal, but she continues to rock her body at night. They are not sure if this
habit is dangerous. How can they help her to decrease the rocking?....

(continued on page 217)

Guidelines for Treating Rhythmic Movement Disorder

Most children with RMD do not require treatment. They tend to grow out of the
habit while still toddlers. However, some children may require treatment, for the
following reasons:

1. Underlying medical problems (for example, reflux of acidic stomach
   contents causing pain from heartburn or ear infection waking up your
   child). Your child's doctor can diagnose and treat these problems.

2. Another sleep disorder waking up your child, such as obstructive sleep
   apnea syndrome. For guidelines in treating obstructive sleep apnea
   syndrome, see Part 3, Chapter 9, "Snoring, Apnea, and Hypoventilation."

3. Developmental delay. Your developmentally delayed child may need
   to wear a helmet or use medication temporarily to decrease
   RMD behavior.

There has not been enough research to make any scientific conclusions on the
best treatment for problematic RMD, whether it is with the use of drugs, or
behavioral interventions.

STEP 1: Prevent Injury

You can try to make the sleeping area safer by using padding, but some children will find ways to head-bang on a hard surface despite your efforts to protect them. When your child first starts head-banging or body-rocking, you may want to watch her to reassure yourself that she is not harming herself, but do not interfere or interact with her because this may inadvertently increase the banging or rocking behavior. After you have seen that she is fine, you don't need to check her each time you hear the movement. You should make sure that the crib or bed is tightly fastened because the movement may loosen the hardware. You may need to move the crib or bed away from the bedroom walls.

STEP 2: Decrease Parental Attention to the Behavior

Do not go to your child each time you hear the rocking noise. When your child is body-rocking or head-banging she is usually drowsy, moving from sleep to wake and back, but not asleep. She may be aware of your presence and learn that you will come to her when she makes these movements. Your attention to the behavior could increase it.

case history: Erin (continued)

Erin is a normal healthy, thriving child with a sleep habit of head-banging, but she does not need any specific treatment. However, her parents should continue to ensure that she is obtaining adequate sleep and that they are not unwittingly reinforcing the movement behavior by giving Erin extra attention at night when she is doing this.

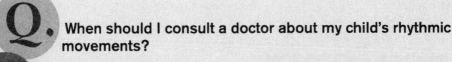

Q. **When should I consult a doctor about my child's rhythmic movements?**

A. Remember that many normal children head-bang and have other types of rhythmic movement disorder. They will likely outgrow the habit by the age of 4 years. These movements may be a method your child has developed to soothe herself to sleep. It is often helpful if you make a video at home of the movement and show this to your doctor if you have any concerns that the movement does not fit the description in this chapter of simple head-banging or body-rocking.

However, see your doctor for further evaluation if the following warning signs arise:

- If your child has a developmental delay, autism, or other neurological problem. Your child may need to wear a helmet to protect himself

- If your child is displaying rhythmic movement during the day while awake and this is interfering with his ability to play

- If your child has harmed himself by the movement

- If you suspect your child has a sleep problem, such as obstructive sleep apnea syndrome

- If you are concerned that the movement is a seizure. If you are able to, make a home video to show your doctor the movement. Your doctor will be able to tell from your description of the movement in most cases if the movement is RMD or a seizure.

Chapter 14

Narcolepsy

CAN YOU IMAGINE what life would be like if you had periodic episodes of irresistible sleep? Can you imagine how this would affect your teenager, at a time in life where being different from the peer group in any way is a burden? If you or your teenager have narcolepsy, sleepiness and the need for naps can overwhelm you at any time — at the dinner table, while talking to friends, at school, or at work.

While normal healthy adults and teenagers experience times of sleepiness like this occasionally, usually related to a few nights of inadequate sleep, people who live with this condition have a chronic problem that varies in severity, but continues throughout life. They can have several different symptoms, but the most prominent one is the irresistible urge to sleep during the day. There are treatments that can reduce, but not always eliminate, the symptoms.

There are many more common causes of excessive sleepiness in children and adolescents, but it is helpful to be aware of this rare cause in order to recognize narcolepsy early and avoid complications, such as academic failure and being stigmatized for needing daytime naps that can accompany this condition. If your child has narcolepsy, he will need to be closely followed by health-care practitioners with specialized expertise in this area.

Did You Know?

Severity of Sleepiness
When children develop narcolepsy, studies show that they are sleepier than adults with this disorder.

What Is Narcolepsy?

Narcolepsy is a rare chronic neurological disorder that affects the regulation of sleep and causes excessive daytime sleepiness. Chronic means that if you have narcolepsy, you will have the condition for your entire lifetime, although the symptoms may be more or less severe at different times in your life. A neurological disorder means that it is caused by a problem related to the nervous system. The main symptom of narcolepsy is excessive daytime sleepiness.

Symptoms of Narcolepsy
Irresistible Naps

A person with narcolepsy will often feel sleepy, regardless of the time of day. There will be times during the day when you have an irresistible urge to nap and after the nap you will feel more awake and alert, but this feeling will not last long. This sleepy feeling will be present during the day even if you have had a long enough period of sleep the previous night. The irresistible naps will occur often when things are quiet or you are bored, but they may also happen at inappropriate times, like while eating, walking or talking. Naps can last from a few minutes to an hour and occur a few times a day.

Abnormal REM

Narcolepsy is also associated with abnormalities of REM (dreaming) sleep. In a normal predictable sleep pattern, you have your first episode of REM sleep 90 to 120 minutes after you fall asleep. In narcolepsy, REM sleep occurs too early in the sleep cycle, which is a sign of a REM abnormality, and the usual characteristics seen during REM sleep are seen during wakefulness. It is like your mind and body are mixed up between sleep and wake. For example, during REM sleep, you have an active, dreaming mind, but your muscles do not have tone, so you do not move. When this sleep state occurs during wakefulness, you may experience the other associated symptoms of narcolepsy — cataplexy (sudden loss of muscle control while awake), hallucinations, and sleep paralysis.

In many people, the sleep attacks will precede the appearance of these REM-associated symptoms, even by decades. The other symptoms (besides excessive sleepiness) may not develop for months to years. When a child is diagnosed with narcolepsy, some parents in retrospect cannot identify exactly when the symptoms started, but believe that their child was sleepier than others his age since early childhood.

REM-Associated Symptoms
Cataplexy

This is the sudden loss of muscle tone. If your child has excessive daytime sleepiness with cataplexy, he likely has narcolepsy. Cataplexy is the one symptom that is very specific to narcolepsy.

Hallucinations

With narcolepsy, you may hallucinate as you fall asleep (called hypnagogic) or as you wake up (hypnopompic). These are vivid dream-like experiences.

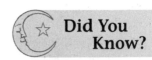

Did You Know?

Cataplexy Facts
Approximately 80% of people with narcolepsy have cataplexy. Research shows that there is a tendency for earlier development of cataplexy in children than in adults, but not in all children. Cataplexy is caused by intense emotional stimulation, such as amusement, surprise, fright, or anger.

CATAPLEXY CHARACTERISTICS

- Loss of voluntary muscle tone, which usually involves both sides of the body.

- Can involve part of the body with the jaw or head or arm dropping, or the whole body completely collapsing.

- Breathing muscles and muscles that control eye movement are not affected.

- Attacks are brief, usually lasting less than a minute, and can recur at varying frequencies from rarely to several times a day.

- There is no change in the level of consciousness during the attack. This means that the person is entirely awake and aware of the cataplexy episode.

- Recovery from the attack is rapid and complete.

Sleep Paralysis

Sleep paralysis is the inability to move or speak for a few seconds to several minutes during the transition between sleep and wakefulness. The episode may be accompanied by a feeling of not being able to breathe. The episode may occur in association with hypnagogic hallucination and be very frightening.

Did You Know?

Narcolepsy Prevalence
The prevalence of narcolepsy varies between ethnic groups:
- In the United States, the prevalence is 2 to 5 per 10,000 people
- In Europe, the prevalence is 3 to 5 per 10,000 people
- In Japan, the prevalence is 1 per 600 people
- Males and females are affected equally

Other Related Symptoms

With narcolepsy, you may also experience disturbed sleep with an increase of nighttime wakings and abnormal behaviors, such as sleepwalking. You may also have episodes of automatic behavior, where you continue to perform a task as you are getting sleepy, like being on 'automatic pilot', and are likely to make an error as you are not alert and fully awake.

Symptom Onset

The symptoms of narcolepsy can start in the teenage years, around 15 years of age, but may not be recognized. In 70% to 80% of people, the symptoms start before the age of 25 years. Studies asking people with narcolepsy to look back and estimate when their symptoms started suggest that 50% of people developed symptoms before 15 years of age and 4.5% say before 5 years of age. Studies report that mean delays between the beginning of symptoms and the time of the diagnosis are 16 to 22 years.

Causes of Narcolepsy

The cause of narcolepsy is complex. Genetic factors are important, but there are also environmental factors (which are not completely understood) that interact with your genetic background to cause narcolepsy. If you have a close family member (such as your mother, father, or siblings) with narcolepsy, the chances that you will have it are small (1% to 2%) but 10 to 40 times greater than people without this family history. There is a genetic marker common in people who have both narcolepsy and cataplexy. However, this genetic marker is not specific for narcolepsy and is also found in 10% to 35% of people who are healthy and do not have this disorder. Most people who are diagnosed with narcolepsy do not have a family member with this condition, and the cause is unknown.

There has been recent research showing that there is a chemical in the brain (called hypocretin/orexin) that is decreased in some people with narcolepsy. This chemical substance is used to transmit signals between brain cells in the parts of the brain that control the symptoms of narcolepsy. In rare cases of narcolepsy, there are some other abnormal processes in the brain, such as trauma or cancer, causing symptoms of narcolepsy.

Other Conditions

Other causes for children to have excessive sleepiness or conditions resembling narcolepsy are seizures, fainting (which can be mistaken for cataplexy), and side effects of other medication.

COMPLICATIONS OF NARCOLEPSY

Major Complications

There are several recognizable complications that you should be aware of if your child or teenager has narcolepsy:

- Accidents due to sleepiness or cataplexy
- Difficulty with attention, concentration, memory, inability to complete assignments on time, or take tests, all leading to academic problems
- Social isolation, absenteeism, dropping out of school
- Depression and other mood disorders
- Loss of academic or vocational opportunities
- Medication side effects
- Stress and family difficulties from the experience of having a sleepy child in the home with special requirements for sleep that impact family activities
- Loss of time for normal childhood experiences and learning due to this increased requirement for sleep

Other Complications

Other complications arise when children with narcolepsy try to conceal their sleepiness from their friends and teachers:

- May mask sleepiness to avoid being punished for being sleepy in class and to avoid social stigmata of being sleepy

- Embarrassment of being sleepy, and/or the cataplexy and being 'different' from other children may lead to social isolation and decreased participation in school and extracurricular activities

- Refusal to participate in sports because excitement will provoke cataplexy

case study: Chantelle

Chantelle is an 18-year-old who was diagnosed with narcolepsy at 17. She came to our sleep clinic because her symptoms are changing. She has recently had her first episode of cataplexy, which frightened her.

When she first met with us a year ago, Chantelle gave us a clear history of her problem, starting at the beginning of junior high. She became gradually sleepier over several months and started to have trouble paying attention at school. Previously, she had been a very good student, but because of her difficulty concentrating and sleepiness, her grades began to drop. She did not see her doctor to discuss these problems, and her parents thought that she was just not trying hard enough at school. Slowly, she became withdrawn and began to miss out not only on schoolwork, but also on social outings with friends.

By Grade 9, Chantelle decided to quit school, to the dismay of her parents, and for a year stayed home, where she was able to sleep and wake on her own schedule. She is now working at a printing press, where the noise, activity and being on her feet during the day help her to stay awake.

She first saw a doctor about her condition only a year ago. He ruled out other problems and referred her to our sleep clinic after being diagnosed with narcolepsy. Chantelle and her parents met with our whole team – doctor, nurse, and social worker – to learn more about narcolepsy. She was referred to an informative Internet site with contact information for the National Narcolepsy Association. She learned about the importance of good sleep hygiene, keeping a regular schedule, and allowing herself opportunities for naps during the day. We also discussed driving, and at that time advised Chantelle not to go for lessons. She was started on a low dose of modafinil, an alerting agent to help her stay awake.

Now she is back at the clinic because she is frightened about this new development of symptoms. She knew all about cataplexy from her reading, but the first time it happened, it was quite scary. She was playing baseball and was at bat. Just as she was about to swing the bat, she felt an overwhelming floppiness and sank to the ground. Luckily, she dropped the bat, and the ball did not hit her. After a few minutes, she was able to get up and resume the game, but she has not played baseball since, and doesn't know if she will ever be able to again....

(continued page 225)

Guidelines for Treating Narcolepsy

STEP 1: Understand the Behavioral Symptoms

Education is a fundamental treatment of narcolepsy. Children, parent, siblings, teachers, coaches, friends, and caregivers need to understand the behavioral symptoms of narcolepsy.

Parents

For parents, this involves:

- Managing the schedule of your child or adolescent to allow for planned regular naps in a non-stigmatized environment at home, school, or work
- Ensuring a regular sleep-wake schedule and adequate nighttime sleep. The schedule needs to be adjusted to be appropriate to the age and developmental stage of your child
- Improving sleep hygiene to ensure restful sleep
- Ensuring your child exercises regularly
- Helping your child avoid stimuli, if possible, that provoke cataplexy
- Helping your child avoid sedentary leisure activities if she is unable to maintain wakefulness
- Being aware of risks involved in dangerous sports and other activities due to sleepiness

Teachers

Teachers need to be educated about this disorder and be aware that your child may have the following problems at school:

- Difficulty with attention, concentration, and memory, which can lead to academic problems

- Difficulty completing assignments on time
- Deterioration of performance on longer tests, but able to show better performance at the beginning of the test before excessive sleepiness interferes
- Need for scheduled naps at school

Adolescents

In addition, adolescents need to be educated about:
- Safe driving practices
- Appropriate career choices
- Possible exacerbation of symptoms with alcohol
- Avoidance of nonprescription drugs

STEP 2: Use Medications

There are specific medications used for the different symptoms of narcolepsy. These include stimulant and non-stimulant medications with alerting effects for the excessive daytime sleepiness, antidepressants, as well as other new medications for cataplexy and the other symptoms of narcolepsy, and medications used to promote more continuous nighttime sleep. Your doctor will provide you with more information on medications when they are prescribed for your child.

Q. **How do I know if my child has narcolepsy?**

A. If you suspect your child has narcolepsy, you need to discuss your concerns with your child's doctor. He will listen to your concerns, ask you questions about your child, conduct a physical examination, and order any blood work or other tests that are needed to rule out other medical problems.

If your child's doctor is concerned about narcolepsy, he will arrange a test in a sleep laboratory to look for signs of narcolepsy. The test requires your child to sleep in the sleep laboratory all night. The next day a daytime test will be done to see how tired your child is and to look for the presence of dreaming sleep in his daytime naps. This test cannot be applied to children under the age of 6 to 7 years of age (when narcolepsy is extremely rare) because it is difficult to evaluate young children in a sleep laboratory. We do not know if children at this young age will display their natural sleepiness or be unable to fall asleep in an unfamiliar environment.

case study: **Chantelle** (continued)

In the clinic, we reviewed Chantelle's sleep hygiene, sleep schedule, and her use of modafinil. It appeared that she was on the correct dose because she was able to stay awake at her job and participate in some social activities in the early evening. We talked about the cataplexy and how to avoid these episodes. Cataplexy cannot always be avoided because it can occur with any emotional excitement. If the episodes continue and are interfering with Chantelle's daily activities, she will be given medication to prevent them .

We discussed with Chantelle safety issues and activities that should be avoided in case she has cataplexy. She is reluctant to continue to play baseball, but is going to try another sport, such as cross-country running, which she also enjoys. For now, Chantelle is not going to get her driver's license. When she decides that her symptoms are well controlled, then she will return to the sleep laboratory for an overnight sleep study and daytime wakefulness study. During the daytime study, Chantelle has to avoid sleeping several times during the day while sitting in a quiet room in the sleep laboratory. This test is one way of determining if a person with narcolepsy is adequately treated to stay awake while driving. During the next few months, Chantelle did have occasional cataplexy, but she did not want to start taking a new medication.

Chapter 15

Teenage Sleepiness

WHAT IS THE DIFFERENCE between teenage sleepiness and sleeplessness? Some teenagers have both — that is, their sleeplessness at bedtime or through the night causes their daytime sleepiness. Less often, teenagers may have sleepiness during the day without being sleepless at night. For example, if your teenager has symptoms of narcolepsy or other increased requirement for sleep, he may have daytime sleepiness, but not nighttime sleeplessness.

Your teenager may be excessively sleepy during the day because of insufficient sleep, the most common sleep problem among adolescents. The cause of his insufficient sleep may be due to difficulty falling asleep from a delayed sleep phase syndrome or other sleep disturbance. Still other teenagers will have the desire to go to sleep but remain sleepless, a frustrating adult condition called primary insomnia, which can begin in late childhood and adolescence.

What Is Teenage Sleepiness?

If your teenager has excessive sleepiness from any cause, this will result in some type of difficulty in his daytime functioning and may include the following symptoms:

- Falling asleep during the day or in class

- Need for a daytime nap

- Difficulty in waking in time for work or school

- Missing activities due to need for sleep

- Drop in grades

- Problems with memory, mood, behavior, attention, or learning in addition to feelings of sleepiness

- Use of caffeine or other stimulant substances in an effort to self-medicate and stay awake

HOW SLEEPY ARE YOU?

Sometimes it is hard to understand the difference between fatigue and sleepiness. Your teenager may be tired during the day, but how likely is it that she will fall asleep?

Epworth Sleepiness Scale

The Epworth sleepiness scale was developed for use by doctors when caring for patients and for use in research studies to quantify sleepiness.

Ask your teenager to complete this questionnaire to see how sleepy she is. You will see by the last questions that this scale was developed for adults who drive and may drink alcohol after lunch; however, you can use it to get an idea about your teenager's sleepiness.

Instructions

How likely are you to doze off or fall asleep in the following situations, in contrast to just feeling tired? This refers to your usual way of life in recent times. Even if you have not done some of these things recently, try to work out how they would have affected you.

Scale

Use the following scale to choose the most appropriate number for each situation.

0 = no chance of dozing
1= slight chance of dozing
2 = moderate chance of dozing
3= high chance of dozing

Situation	Chance of dozing
Sitting and reading	
Watching television	
Sitting inactive in a public place (a theater or meeting)	
Riding as a passenger in a car for an hour	
Lying down to rest in the afternoon	
Sitting and talking to someone	
Sitting quietly after lunch without alcohol	
Driving a car while stopped for a few minutes in traffic	
Total Score	

Score

A total score of more than 11 suggests a high probability of a sleep problem. You should arrange for your teenager to discuss this with your doctor.

What Are the Causes of Excessive Sleepiness in Teenagers?

The most common causes of sleepiness in teenagers are insufficient sleep, disturbed sleep, or an increased requirement for sleep.

Insufficient Sleep

The most common cause of sleepiness is insufficient sleep. This may be due to getting to bed too late, having an irregular schedule, or having difficulty with falling asleep or early morning waking from a delayed or (rarely) an advanced sleep phase, for example. Some of these causes are within their own control, such as having too many social, school, and work commitments, or staying up late at night playing on the computer, talking on the telephone, or watching television.

Disturbed Sleep

Insufficient sleep is not the only possible factor in causing excessive sleepiness. Other factors may disturb sleep and result in daytime sleepiness.

Signs of Insufficient Sleep

Teenager may notice	Parent may notice	Teacher may notice
Able to concentrate better in the morning	Need for daytime naps	Learning, memory, or behavior problems
Able to start the beginning of tests or assignments, but be not able to complete them	Falls asleep easily in passive situations (for example, watching television or driving in the car)	Fluctuating levels of attention
Lack of energy to participate in school and extracurricular activities	Missing school or extracurricular activities because he is "too tired" to attend	May mistakenly feel that student is not motivated or unable to do work, rather than sleepy
Feelings of anger or frustration caused by his sleepiness	Frustration with the teenager's need for sleep felt by other family members	Adolescent sleepiness may be noticed, but mistakenly attributed to use of drugs or alcohol

- Sleep disorders, such as sleep apnea, frequent nightmares, or restless legs syndrome
- Mood or psychological problems (for example, depression)
- Use of or withdrawal from drugs or alcohol
- Medical problems (for example, pain from any cause)
- Side effects of drugs prescribed for another medical problem

Increased Requirement for Sleep

- Narcolepsy
- Other rare syndromes that cause a need for increased sleep

What is Primary Insomnia?

Some teenagers develop an adult type of insomnia, where they try to get adequate sleep but can't. If this is the case, your teenager may have difficulty falling asleep or staying asleep, which leads to impairment in daytime. If your teenager is really trying to get to sleep, has improved his sleep hygiene and schedule, and is not able to sleep, he may have primary insomnia.

WHAT THE TEXTBOOKS SAY

Primary insomnia is characterized by the following features:

- Your teenager has difficulty falling or staying asleep, or his sleep does not restore his energy normally. These problems must have been occurring for at least a month to be classified as primary insomnia.

- This disturbance to your teenager's sleep or the fatigue that it causes during the day causes significant distress or a problem in his daily functioning at school, work, or with friends or family.

- This condition is called primary insomnia because it is not secondary to another problem – psychiatric, medical, or sleep disorder – and it is not due to the effects of taking any prescription, nonprescription, or street drugs.

(Based on the International Classification of Sleep Disorders, 2001)

Primary Insomnia Factors

Everyone has occasional sleepless nights, but what causes this to become a chronic problem? A possible answer rests in the interaction of three factors:

Predisposing factors: Everyone has some predisposition to have disturbed sleep. Your teenager's tendency to develop insomnia may run in your family. Another possible problem may be with hyperarousal, predisposing to insomnia.

Precipitating factors: The precipitant of this problem can be many different factors. If you are predisposed to insomnia, it may be triggered by a circumstance (sleeping in a hotel room, for example) that for someone with a low predisposition to insomnia would not be problematic.

Perpetuating factors: In the definition of primary insomnia, it must last for at least 1 month, so there have to be circumstances that continue or perpetuate the problem. These circumstances can include poor sleep habits, an erratic sleep/wake schedule, or being excessively worried about getting enough sleep.

---

case history: **Shannon**

Shannon was 17 years old when she first visited our sleep clinic with her mother, April. Shannon had never been able to fall asleep easily, but recently, she is lying in bed from 11:00 p.m. until 2:00 a.m., often awake and frustrated. This leaves her feeling tired the next day, and she ends up drinking a lot of coffee to stay awake. April recalled that Shannon came home from the hospital as a newborn with her eyes wide open. From day one, she did not like to sleep. Over the years, April (who is a single mother) gave in to Shannon's wakefulness and did not enforce a regular bedtime.

Despite what April has always felt to be inadequate sleep for her daughter, Shannon has done well in school, holds a part-time job at McDonald's, and volunteers at the local community center, where she teaches English to new immigrants. Shannon and April want to know what can be done to help her fall asleep. They are wondering if there is any medicine that she can take? ...

(continued on page 234)

Guidelines for Treating Teenage Sleepiness

TREATMENTS USED FOR insufficient sleep, sleep disturbances, and increased requirement for sleep have been presented in previous chapters. For primary insomnia, the following behavioral-based strategies can be tried, but you may need additional support from your doctor or a counselor to help your teenager make these changes to her sleep habits.

Primary Insomnia

STEP 1: Improve Sleep Hygiene and Establish a Regular Sleep Schedule

With you teenager, review the guidelines for healthy sleep hygiene in Part 1, Chapter 3, "Sleep Hygiene." The following strategies will only work in combination with attention to good sleep habits and a regular schedule.

STEP 2: Use One or a Combination of Behavioral Strategies

There are several effective behavior therapies for treating primary insomnia.

Stimulus Control Therapy

This treatment is based on a theory that when you cannot fall asleep at night, you begin to see bedtime as a frustrating time. This notion then becomes a self-fulfilling prophecy. When you get into bed, you can't fall asleep because you are used to being frustrated. This feeling returns each night.

To change this behavior, stimulus control therapy can be tried in order to teach a more pleasant association with your bedtime and sleeping environment – to 'break the cycle' of frustration. You can assist your teenager with the following steps to control change his bedtime attitude.

Stimulus Control Routine

1. Go to bed only when sleepy. You don't want your teenager to lie in bed for hours feeling frustrated.

2. Only use the bed and bedroom for sleep. This means no television, computer, music, or telephone in the room. Temporarily, your child should even do his homework in a different room.

3. Encourage your child to get out of bed if he can't sleep. If he gets into bed and can't fall asleep within 15 to 20 minutes, he should get out of bed and go into another room, where he should do a quiet, non-stimulating activity, such as reading a book, writing letters, or listening to quiet music, all done sitting up, not lying on the couch,

where he may fall asleep. Do this until he feels sleepy, and then get back into bed. He should repeat this until he falls asleep within 15 to 20 minutes of getting into bed.

④ Get up at the same time every day. Your child should get up at the same time every morning, 7 days a week, even if he was unable to sleep the previous night. This way, he will start to establish a schedule of sleep and wake. He cannot force himself to fall asleep, but he can ensure that he wakes up in the morning. If he does have trouble falling asleep, but still wakes up at the same time, he will be mildly sleep deprived and then more likely to fall asleep at a desired time the next night.

⑤ Don't nap during the day. In general, naps are not a problem if teenagers do not have any sleep difficulties. However, if your child has insomnia and naps during the day, he will be much less likely to resolve the insomnia because he will have less sleep debt at night and less sleep pressure or natural tendency to fall asleep.

Sleep Restriction Therapy

In this therapy, your teenager's time in bed is matched to the time he reports he is able to sleep. This prevents lying in bed sleeplessly. Then the sleep time is gradually lengthened until you get to the desired sleep time.

For example, your teenager may complain of only being able to sleep 5 hours at night. She gets ready for bed with a bedtime routine at 11:00 p.m., and turns off the lights at 12:00. She then experiences extreme frustration, lying in bed and attempting to sleep until around 1:00 a.m., when she finally falls asleep. She wakes spontaneously, even on weekends, around 6:00 a.m., and even when she desires to sleep later, she cannot do so. She becomes convinced that she only sleeps 5 hours per night.

To reduce this feeling of frustration and lengthen your child's sleep period, you can help her with the following sleep restriction strategies. The goal is for child to obtain the amount of sleep that she needs to not feel tired during the day.

Sleep Restriction Routine

Explain to your teenager that you want her to be sleeping for at least 90% of the time that she is actually in her bed. If she feels that she is only sleeping 5 hours, tell her to be in bed only for 5 hours and 30 minutes. This way, if she is only sleeping 5 hours, she will only be awake in bed for 30 minutes. In this example, she should go to bed at 12:30 a.m. and get out of bed at 6:00 a.m.

Follow this strategy for 4 to 7 days. She will become more tired because she is mildly sleep deprived; however, she should not feel much different than before because her initial problem was that she could only sleep for 5 hours. She now has the opportunity to sleep for 5.5 hours.

For the next 4 to 7 nights, encourage your child to go to bed at 12:00 and get out of bed at 6:00 a.m. If she is able to fall asleep by 12:30, then she will be sleeping for 5.5 out of 6 hours of being in bed, which is still about 90% of the time that she is in bed. Once she is sleeping at least 5.5 hours for 4 nights in a row, then you go to the next step.

For the next 4 to 7 nights, encourage her to go to bed at 11:30 p.m. and try to sleep for at least 6 hours.

Continue this pattern of gradually increasing the time that she is in bed, provided she is sleeping at least 90% of the time that she is actually in bed. She should only increase her time in bed when she has slept 90% of the time for 4 nights in a row.

For this strategy to work effectively, your teenager should keep a consistent morning wake-up time and not nap during the day.

Relaxation Therapies

Relaxation therapies can be used to decrease the high level of arousal that some people with insomnia feel (often both during the daytime and at night). These methods may be useful for a motivated adolescent, but they require regular practice. In addition, you would need to discuss these with your health-care provider and likely have someone who is trained in these techniques teach them to your teenager. These are not the type of therapies that you can easily learn from a self-help book.

Progressive muscle relaxation

Your child learns to tense and relax muscles systematically in a repetitive manner.

Biofeedback

Your child learns how to relax some aspect of the body (for example, muscle tension) by using sound (auditory) or sight (visual) feedback.

Imagery training

Your child learns to focus on a pleasant or neutral image in order to relax and reduce tension.

Thought stopping

Your child learns to relax by not allowing worrisome thoughts or concerns at night.

Behavioral Treatments with Sleeping Pills

In some cases, your doctor will recommend combining behavioral strategies for insomnia with a short course of sleeping medications. For instance, your doctor may suggest that your teenager takes the sleeping medication at the beginning of treatment in combination with the behavioral strategies to break the cycle of frustration from not sleeping. However, the most effective way to resolve this type of insomnia is with behavioral methods, not pills. In most cases, your teenager, if motivated to improve his sleep, will be able to improve his sleep without sleeping medication.

Q. **When should I consult a doctor about my teenager's sleepiness?**

A. Consult with your health-care provider if you have concerns about the following problems or any other persistent worrisome symptoms:

- If there is a change in his sleep pattern or feeling of daytime sleepiness that does not resolve using behavioral strategies

- If you are concerned that there is an underlying problem with his medical health, mood, behavior, learning, attention, alcohol, or other substance abuse

- If there is a drop in school grades

- If there are any signs of breathing problems during sleep, as described in Part 3, Chapter 9, "Snoring, Apnea, and Hypoventilation"

- If your teenager has a drowsy-driving accident

- If your teenager is falling asleep during the day or in class

case history: **Shannon** (continued)

After thorough review of Shannon's case in the clinic, we were able to eliminate anxiety, stress, and depression as causes of her sleepiness, and determined that Shannon had primary insomnia. She was instructed to pay attention to sleep hygiene, especially to developing a regular sleep schedule, waking at the same time each morning. She had never done this since infancy. We explained the limited role for sleeping pills and their possible adverse effects in treating primary insomnia in adolescents.

April took Shannon's computer, telephone, cellphone, MP3 player, and television out of her room. The room was designated for sleeping only. On her own, Shannon cut back on her caffeine consumption slowly and then eliminated caffeine from her diet altogether. She tried the stimulus control suggestions to decrease her frustration with not being able to fall asleep at night.

During the next 6 months, Shannon was able to recognize a marked improvement in her ability to fall asleep. She was also happy to notice more energy during the day and a better ability to concentrate on her schoolwork. April reported that, although Shannon would not admit it, she was much easier to get along with at home.

The use of behavioral strategies was effective in helping Shannon to deal with her insomnia, though both April and Shannon are now aware that this can be an ongoing problem. They know they have to continue to pay attention to the importance of good sleep.

Chapter 16

Sleep During Pregnancy

L ET'S TAKE A STEP back and review sleep during pregnancy. A retrospective look at your sleep habits while pregnant may help you cope with your baby's sleep pattern as a newborn and also help prepare you for your next pregnancy, if you choose to have another child.

Women have different experiences of being pregnant. If your health is good, you may experience pregnancy as a period of happiness and anticipation. However, there are many challenges during pregnancy, and for some, it is not such an easy go. Whatever else happens during pregnancy, you are likely to experience disrupted sleep and daytime fatigue. While most pregnant women cope well with lack of sleep, others don't. You need to take sleep problems during pregnancy seriously because they may have consequences for your developing fetus, as well as for yourself. Sleep disruption does not, of course, end when your baby is born. Any ongoing sleep problems will affect you detrimentally, and, therefore, may affect your interactions with your child.

What Are Common Sleep Problems during Pregnancy?

Pregnancy significantly affects both the quantity and quality of your sleep during all trimesters:

During the first trimester:

- You may feel that the quality of your sleep decreases and the number of times you wake during the night increases.
- You may notice you are more sleepy during the day.

During the second trimester:

- You may notice that your sleep seems more normal, although one in five pregnant women during the second trimester still continue to have problems with sleep and daytime fatigue.

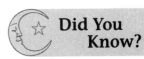

Did You Know?

Postpartum Depression
Sleep disruption that results from caring for a new baby can play an important role in the development or recurrence of postpartum psychiatric illness in the mother. We don't know for sure that they cause sleep problems in the child. If you are feeling depressed, you may not be able to attend properly to your baby's sleep hygiene.

Did You Know?

Pregnancy Sleep Problem Prevalence
In a survey conducted by The National Sleep Foundation in the United States in 2003, more than half the women surveyed reported sleep disturbance during pregnancy, and 70% of these women reported that it interfered with daily functioning on at least a few days a month. Although this survey was limited by some factors, such as not including young pregnant women under the age of 30 years, it still provides valuable information on the frequency of pregnancy-associated sleep problems.

During the third trimester:

- You may notice worsening insomnia, increased daytime sleeping, and decreased alertness.

- Toward the end of pregnancy, you have an increased release of the hormone oxytocin during the night. This causes contractions of your uterus in preparation for birth, but may also cause you to be uncomfortable at night and disrupt your sleep.

- You will need to urinate more frequently, and you may experience discomfort in the abdomen or back, as well as leg cramps and heartburn, and feel your fetus moving when you are trying to sleep.

Developing Sleep Disorders during Pregnancy

Sleep disturbance during pregnancy is very common. Although you may have never had a sleep disorder, you may experience one during your pregnancy for the first time. In addition, if you do have a mild sleep disorder, the symptoms may worsen during pregnancy. Insomnia associated with obstructive sleep apnea syndrome (OSAS), restless legs syndrome (RLS), and primary insomnia (with no clear cause) may appear or worsen during pregnancy.

FACTORS CONTRIBUTING TO DISRUPTED SLEEP IN PREGNANCY

- Hormonal/endocrine changes, such as increased progesterone and prolactin levels (progesterone makes you drowsy)

- Increased size

- Fetal movement

- Bladder distension

- Nausea and vomiting

- Body temperature fluctuations

- Anything that disturbs sleep in general in adults can also affect your sleep during pregnancy, such as medications, sleep disorders, and psychiatric or medical illness

Obstructive Sleep Apnea Syndrome

In adults, OSAS is most common in men, especially those who are overweight, and in postmenopausal women. It is rare in non-pregnant women of reproductive age probably because progesterone, a reproductive hormone that decreases after menopause, works to stimulate breathing in younger women. However, your risk of having OSAS increases significantly if you are both pregnant and overweight. There has not been enough research in this area to know how common this problem is during pregnancy.

POSSIBLE CONSEQUENCES OF OSAS FOR THE FETUS AND BABY

While there has not been enough research yet to determine whether or not the drop in your oxygen levels caused by OSAS during sleep will affect your fetus, a small number of studies have suggested several serious possible consequences in pregnancy:

- Pregnancy-induced high blood pressure

- Problems for the baby at the time of birth with need for help with breathing

- Obstructive sleep apnea syndrome combined with other problems of pregnancy, such as obesity and diabetes mellitus, may result in fetal growth problems

You should talk to your health-care provider about the risk of having sleep problems like OSAS if you are pregnant, overweight or have a large neck size with any of the following symptoms:

- Snore during sleep

- Wake with morning headaches

- Feel excessive daytime fatigue

Restless Legs Syndrome

You may have symptoms of RLS before pregnancy that worsen enough to be recognized while you are pregnant. This may be related to lower iron stores during pregnancy and a family history of RLS, which makes you more prone to develop it during pregnancy.

You may experience leg cramps while you are awake and daytime sleepiness or fatigue. Your partner may notice or complain that you kick when you are sleeping.

POSSIBLE CONSEQUENCES OF RLS FOR THE FETUS AND BABY

If you have been diagnosed with RLS during pregnancy, you may wonder if there are any adverse effects for your fetus or newborn. Although there has been some research in the effect of OSAS on the fetus, there are no specific studies on the effects of RLS during pregnancy. However, anything that disrupts your sleep and increases your fatigue during pregnancy, including RLS, has the potential to affect your energy level in the post-partum period.

Insomnia

Insomnia may appear for the first time or become more pronounced during pregnancy. You may find that you have trouble falling asleep, staying asleep, and waking too early in the morning. For you, insomnia may put you at greater risk for developing depression. If your sleep is disrupted by insomnia or another sleep problem during pregnancy and in the weeks after your baby is born, you are likely to be at higher risk for developing a postpartum mood disorder. If you already have a mood disorder, you may experience an increase in the symptoms triggered by sleep deprivation related to pregnancy.

POSSIBLE CONSEQUENCES OF INSOMNIA FOR THE FETUS AND BABY

Pregnant women commonly use over-the-counter remedies, alcohol, and prescription drugs to treat their insomnia. In a National Sleep Foundation survey of pregnant women (1998), 7% were found to use over-the counter medications, 7% used alcohol at some point in the pregnancy, 4% used prescription medications for this purpose. These types of sleep aids during pregnancy could have significant consequences for the developing baby. For example, it is not known if there is a safe threshold for alcohol during pregnancy, and even small amounts taken to help fall asleep are potentially harmful to your developing fetus.

In addition, disrupted sleep during pregnancy and in the early postpartum period can affect how you feel emotionally, function during the day, remember, think, and perform tasks, making those that are easy seem difficult — symptoms that have consequences for how you care for your child, including her own sleep behavior. Significantly, insomnia affects your ability to realize how your own sleepiness is impacting your performance.

Guidelines for Treating Sleep Disorders in Pregnancy

Obstructive Sleep Apnea Syndrome

The treatment for OSAS is different for children than for pregnant women. The usual treatment for your child if he has OSAS is to have his tonsils and adenoids removed, whereas if the mother has OSAS during pregnancy, it can be treated with a machine providing continuous positive airway pressure (CPAP) during sleep. This treatment has been shown to be safe during pregnancy. If your problem with breathing is only mild, you may only need simple changes, such as sleeping on your side.

Restless Legs Syndrome

There are several safe and effective physical and nutritional therapies for RLS:

1. Massage and stretch the leg muscles
2. Take a warm bath in the evening before going to sleep
3. Wear support stockings on your legs in bed
4. Take an iron supplement if your iron stores in your blood are low (this needs to be checked by your doctor)
5. Your doctor may prescribe medications if the problem is severe.

Insomnia

Sleep hygiene is important for everyone, but especially for pregnant women and new mothers.

STEP 1: Improve Sleep Hygiene

1. Establish a regular sleep/wake schedule. This will be more difficult after the baby's arrival, but it is possible if your partner or others can help out.
2. Avoid caffeinated food and beverages, especially in the afternoon and evening.
3. Reduce the amount of fluids that you drink in the evening.
4. Make sure that the temperature in your bedroom is comfortable.
5. Consider a nap in the daytime. Some women find that having a nap in the daytime is helpful, whereas others find that it affects nighttime sleep. Each woman must work out what is best for her in this respect.

STEP 2: Decrease Severity of Insomnia Symptoms

1. Try gentle exercise, such as walking and stretching, which can help with sleep.
2. Try relaxation techniques and massage, which have proven to be useful for treating insomnia and are safe during pregnancy.
3. Take a warm bath close to bedtime.
4. Should sleep disruption turn out to be an ongoing problem for you, consider taking a course in cognitive behavioral therapy (CBT) for insomnia, usually led by a psychologist or a psychiatrist. Discuss your options with your health-care provider.

STEP 3: Avoid Complications

1. Panic: Don't panic. Many women experience sleep problems and are able to cope with minimal adverse effects. Sleep usually improves once the baby starts to develop a routine sleep schedule.
2. Despair: Remember that if things get bad, help is available from your doctor, nurse, community, family, and friends.
3. Sleep aids: Do not use alcohol or any over-the-counter medications or herbal preparations to treat insomnia unless you have discussed this with your doctor.
4. Feeling guilty. Do not feel guilty about accepting help, whatever that may be. Remember that the more you take care of yourself, the more you are taking care of your family. Your health is vital to your baby's well-being.

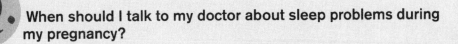

Q. **When should I talk to my doctor about sleep problems during my pregnancy?**

A. Talk to your doctor:

- If you think you are having a sleep problem beyond what would be expected for someone in your situation

- If you are having great difficulty switching your mind off at night and this is making it difficult for you to fall asleep

- If you awaken frequently at night, even though you do not need to go to the washroom

- If you are told by your bed partner that you snore, stop breathing, or kick your legs while asleep.

- If you are taking any medications, either prescribed or over-the-counter, or drinking alcohol in order to asleep. Tell your doctor if you are taking herbal preparations; there is little data regarding the safety and usefulness of these during pregnancy. They should be avoided or used only under the supervision of your doctor.

- If you feel extremely sleepy in the daytime. This is particularly important if you have a history of a mood disorder (for example, depression or bipolar disorder).

- If you live far from family and friends and lack a social support network

- If you think you have poor coping skills and are concerned about the demands that will be placed on you with your newborn baby

- If you are concerned that you may have difficulty adjusting to the new role of being a mother

Your doctor will take a thorough history of your problem, including your pre-pregnancy sleep patterns and history of insomnia or other sleep problems. You may find that just talking aloud about these concerns is helpful in itself.

Your doctor will also make sure that there are no medical causes for your sleep problem. She may check your level of thyroid hormone and iron stores in your blood. If she suspects that you have a sleep disorder, she may refer you for an overnight sleep study in a sleep clinic. Your doctor can listen to your concerns about coping with your newborn. She will be able to help you to contact resources in the community to provide you with support while you are coping with your sleep deprivation, and the excitement and challenges of motherhood.

The outcome should be a mother and a baby who sleep well and enjoy good health.

Resources

Associations and Clinics

American Academy of Pediatrics
141 Northwest Point Boulevard
Elk Grove Village, IL 60007-1098
Tel: (847) 434-4000
Website: www.aap.org
An organization of American pediatricians committed to the well-being of all infants, children, adolescents and young adults. The website contains a parenting corner.

American Academy of Sleep Medicine
One Westbrook Corporate Center, Suite 920
Westchester, IL 60154
Tel: (708) 492-0930
Website: www.aasmnet.org
A professional association dedicated to sleep medicine with information on all aspects of sleep disorders, as well as an educational website: www.sleepeducation.com

American Sleep Apnea Association
1424 K Street NW, Suite 302
Washington, DC 20005
Tel: (202) 293-3650
Website: www.sleepapnea.org
An organization dedicated to reducing injury, disability, and death from sleep apnea and to enhancing the well-being of those affected by sleep apnea.

Canadian Paediatric Society
2305 St. Laurent Boulevard
Ottawa, ON K1G 4J8
Tel.: (613) 526-9397
Website: www.cps.ca
A national advocacy association of Canadian pediatricians committed to the health needs of children and youth. Parent handouts on pediatric topics, including sleep, are available on this website at www.caringforkids.cps.ca

Canadian Sleep Society
Website: www.css.to
A professional association of clinicians, scientists, and technologists dedicated to further the advancement and understanding of sleep and its disorders through scientific study and public awareness. Brochures on sleep disorders are available on the website.

The Hospital for Sick Children
Sleep Clinic and Sleep Laboratory
555 University Avenue
Toronto, ON M5G 1X8
Website: www.sickkids.ca

Narcolepsy Network
79 Main Street
North Kingstown, RI 02852
Tel: (401) 667-2523
Website: www.narcolepsynetwork.org
An American national nonprofit patient support organization for people with narcolepsy (or similar disorders), families, friends, and professionals who are involved in the treatment, research, and public education regarding narcolepsy.

National Sleep Foundation
1522 K Street, NW, Suite 500
Washington, DC 20005
Tel: (202) 347-3471
Website: www.sleepfoundation.org
An independent nonprofit American
organization dedicated to improving public
health and safety, increasing awareness and
understanding of sleep and sleep disorders,
and supporting education, research, and
advocacy. The website has information for
the public.

Restless Legs Syndrome Foundation
819 Second Street SW
Rochester, MN 55902-2985
Tel: (507) 287-6465
Website: www.rls.org
An organization dedicated to improving
the lives of the men, women, and children
who live with this often devastating disease.
The organization's goals are to increase
awareness of restless legs syndrome (RLS),
to improve treatments, and through
research, to find a cure.

Print Resources

Healthy Sleep Habits, Happy Child
by Marc Weissbluth
New York, NY: Random House Publishing
Group, 2003

**Helping Your Child Sleep Through
the Night**
by Joanne Cuthbertson & Susie Schevill
New York, NY: Broadway Books, 2002

In Search of Sleep
by Bonny Reichert
Toronto, ON: Key Porter Books, 2001

**Sleep Better: A Guide to Improving
Sleep for Children with Special Needs**
by V. Mark Durand
Baltimore, MD: Paul H. Brookes Publishing
Co., 1998

Sleeping Like a Baby
by Avi Sadeh
New Haven, CT: Yale University Press, 2001

Sleeping Through the Night
by Jodi A Mindell
New York, NY: Harper Collins Publishers,
Inc., 1997

Solve Your Child's Sleep Problems
by Richard Ferber
New York, NY: Simon & Schuster, Inc., 2006

Take Charge of Your Child's Sleep
by Judy A. Owens and Jody A Mindell
New York, NY: Marlowe & Co., 2005

The No-Cry Sleep Solution
by Elizabeth Pantley
New York, NY: Contemporary Books, 2002

References

Adams SM, Jones DR, Esmail A, Mitchell EA. What affects the age of the first sleeping through the night? J. Paediatar. Child Health 2004;40:96–101.

Allen RP, Picchietti D, Hening W, Trenkwalder C,Walters AS, Montplaisir J. Restless legs syndrome: diagnostic criteria, special considerations and epidemiology. Sleep Medicine 2003;4:101–19.

Aloia MS, Arnedt JT, Davis JD, et al. Neuropsychological sequelae of obstructive sleep apnea-hypopnea syndrome: a critical review. Journal of the International Neuropsychological Society 2004;10:772–85.

American Academy of Sleep Medicine. International Classification of Sleep Disorders, Revised: Diagnostic and Coding Manual. Chicago, IL: American Academy of Sleep Medicine, 2001.

Anders TF. Infant sleep, nighttime relationships, and attachment. Psychiatry 1994;57(1):11–20.

Banerjee D, Vitiello, Grunstein RR. Pharmacotherapy for excessive daytime sleepiness. Sleep Medicine Reviews 2004;8:339–54.

Barr, RG, Paterson, JA, MacMartin, LM, Lehtonen, L, Young, SN. Prolonged and unsoothable crying bouts in infants with and without colic. Dev Beh Ped 2005;26(1):14–23.

Bootzin RR, Stevens SJ. Adolescents, substance abuse, and the treatment of insomnia and daytime sleepiness. Clinical Psychology Review 2005;25:629–44.

Burnham MM, Goodlin-Jones BL, Gaylor EE, Anders TF. Nighttime sleep-wake patterns and self-soothing from birth to one year of age: A longitudinal intervention study. Journal of Child Psychology and Psychiatry 2002;43(6):713–25.

Caldwell PH, Edgar D, Hodson E, et al. Bedwetting and toileting problems in children. Medical Journal of Australia 2005;182(4):190–95.

Carskadon MA, Acebo C, Jenni OG. Regulation of adolescent sleep. Implications for behavior. Ann. N.Y. Acad. Sci 2004;1021:276–91.

Carskadon MA, Acebo CA. Regulation of sleepiness in adolescence: Updates insights, and speculation. Sleep 2002;25(6):606–14.

Carskadon MA, Labyak SE, Acebo C et al. Intrinsic circadian period of adolescent humans measured in conditions of forced desynchrony. Neuroscience Letters 1999;260:129–32.

Carskadon MA, Viera C, Acebo C. Association between puberty and delayed phase preference. Sleep 1993;16:258–62.

Chervin RD, Archbold KH, Dillon JE, Panahi P, Pituch KJ, Dahl RE, Guilleminault C. Inattention, hyperactivity, and symptoms of sleep-disordered breathing. Pediatrics 2002;109:449–56.

Christer H, Jaakko K, Markku P, Markku K. Parasomnias: co-occurrence and genetics. Psychiatric Genetics 2001;11(2):65–70.

Cooper J, Tyler L. Wallace I et al. No evidence of sleep apnea in children with attention deficit hyperactivity disorder. Clinical Pediatrics 2004;43(7):609–14.

D'cruz O, Vaughn BV. Parasomnias: An update. Seminars in Pediatric Neurology 2001;8(4):251–57.

Dagan Y. Circadian rhythm sleep disorders. Sleep Medicine Reviews 2002;6(1):45–55.

Davis KF, Parker KP, Montgomery GL. Sleep in infants and young children: part one: normal sleep. J Pediatr Health Care 2004;18:65–71.

De Laat A, Macaluso GM. Sleep bruxism as a motor disorder. Movement Disorders 2002;17(supp 2):S67–69.

Eckerberg B, Treatment of sleep problems in families with young children: effects of treatment in family well-being. Acta Paediatr 2004;93:126–34.

Edwards N, Middleton PG, Blyton DM, Sullivan CE. Sleep disorder breathing and pregnancy. Thorax. 2002:555–58.

Etzioni T, Katz N, Hering E, Ravd S, Pillar G. Controlled sleep restriction for rhythmic movement disorder 2005;147:393–95.

Fallone G, Owens JA, Deane J. Sleepiness in children and adolescents: Clinical implications. Sleep Medicine Reviews 2002;6(4):287–306.

Fehlings D, Weiss S, Stephens D. Frequent night awakenings in preschool children referred to a sleep disorders clinic: The role of non-adaptive sleep associations. Children's Health Care 2001;30:43–55.

Feldman M. and Community Paediatrics Committee. Management of primary nocturnal enuresis. Paediatrics & Child Health 2005;10(10):611–614.

Ferber R, Kryger M. Principles and practice of sleep medicine in the child. Philadelphia, PA: W.B. Saunders Co., 1995.

France KG, Blampied NM. Infant sleep disturbance: Description of a problem behaviour process. Sleep Medicine Reviews 1999;3(4):265–80.

Garcia J, Rosen G, Mahowald M. Circadian rhythms and circadian rhythm disorders in children and adolescents. Seminars in Pediatric Neurology 2001;8(4):229–40.

Garcia J, Wills L. Sleep disorders in children and teens. Postgrad Med 2000;107(3):161–78.

Gibson, ES, Powles ACP, Thabane L, O'Brien, S, Molnar DS, Trajanovic N, et al. Sleepiness is serious in adolescence: Two surveys of 3235 Canadian students. BMC Public Health 2006;6;116:1–9

Givan DC. The sleepy child. The Pediatric Clinics of North America 2004;51(1):15–32.

Glaze D. Childhood insomnia: Why Chris can't sleep. The Pediatric Clinics of North America 2004;51(1):33–50.

Glazener CMA, Evans JHC, Peto RE. Alarm interventions for nocturnal enuresis in children. The Cochrane Database of Systematic Reviews 2003, Issue 2. Art. No.: CD002911. DOI: 10.1002/14651858.CD002911.

Glazener CMA, Evans JHC, Peto RE. Complex behavioural and educational interventions for nocturnal enuresis in children. The Cochrane Database of Systematic Reviews 2004, Issue 1. Art. No.: CD004668. DOI: 10.1002/14651858.CD004668.

Glazener CMA, Evans JHC, Peto RE. Tricyclic and related drugs for nocturnal enuresis in children. The Cochrane Database of Systematic Reviews 2003, Issue 3. Art. No.: CD002117. DOI: 10.1002/14651858.CD002117.

Glazener CMA, Evans JHC. Desmopressin for nocturnal enuresis in children. The Cochrane Database of Systematic Reviews 2002 Issue 3. Art. No.: CD002112. DOI: 10.1002/14651858.CD002112. [Amended: 25 May 2004].

Glazener CMA, Evans JHC. Simple behavioural and physical interventions for nocturnal enuresis in children. The Cochrane Database of Systematic Reviews 2004, Issue 2. Art. No.: CD003637.pub2. DOI: 10.1002/14651858.CD003637.pub2.

Goodlin-Jones BL, Burnham MM, Gaylor EE, Anders TF. Night waking, sleep-wake organization, and self-soothing in the first year of life. Jn of Developmental & Behavioral Pediatrics 2001;22(4):226–33.

Goodman DS, Brodie C, Ayida GA. Restless leg syndrome in pregnancy. Br Med J 1988;29:1101–02.

Gottlieb DJ, Vezina RM, Chase C, Lesko Sm, Heeren TC, Weese-Mayer DE et al. Symptoms of sleep-disordered breathing in 5-year-old children are associated with sleepiness and problem behaviors. Pediatrics 2003;112(3):870–77.

Gozal D, Pope DW Jr. Snoring during early childhood and academic performance at ages thirteen to fourteen years. Pediatrics 2001;107:1394–99.

Guilleminault C, Lee JH, Chan A. Pediatric Obstructive Sleep Apnea Syndrome. Arch Pediatr Adolesc Med 2005;159:775–85.

Guilleminault C, Palombini L, Pelayo R, Chervin RD. Sleepwalking and sleep terrors in prepurbertal children: what triggers them? Pediatrics 2003;111(1): e17–25.

Guilleminault C. Disorders of arousal in children: Somnambulism and night terrors. Sleep and Its Disorders in Children. New York, NY: C. Raven Press, 1987:243–52.

Hauck FR. Olanrewaju O, Siadaty MS. Do pacifiers reduce the risk of sudden infant death syndrome? A meta-analysis. Pediatrics 2005;116(5):e716–e723.

Heussler HS. Common causes of sleep disruption and daytime sleepiness: childhood sleep disorders II. Medical Journal of Australia 2005;182(9):484–89.

Hiscock H, Jordan B. Problem crying in infancy. Medical Journal of Australia 2004;181(9):507–12.

Houghton WC, Scammell TE, Thorpy M. Pharmacotherapy for cataplexy. Sleep Medicine Reviews 2004;8:355–66.

Howard BJ, Wong J. Sleep Disorders. Pediatrics in Review 2001;22(10):327–42.

Hublin C, Kaprio J, Partinen M, Heikkila K, Koskenvuo M. Prevalence and genetics of sleepwalking: a population-based twin study. Neurology 1997;48:177–81.

Iglowstein I, Jenni OG, Molinari L, et al. Sleep duration from infancy to adolescence: Reference values and generational trends. Pediatrics 2003;111(2):302–307.

Ivanenko A, Crabtree VM, Tauman R, Gozal D. Melatonin in children and adolescents with insomnia: a retrospective study. Clinical Pediatrics 2003;42(1):51–58.

Ivanenko A, Crabtree VM, Gozal D. Sleep and depression in children and adolescents. Sleep medicine reviews 2005;9:115–29.

Jan JE, Freeman RD. Melatonin therapy for circadian rhythm sleep disorders in children with multiple disabilities: What have we learned in the last decade? Developmental Medicine & Child Neurology 2004;46(11):776–82.

Jenni OG, O'Connor BB. Children's sleep: An interplay between culture and biology. Pediatrics 2005;115:204–16.

Jenni OG, Zinggeler Fuhrer H, Iglowstein I, Molinari L, Largo RH. A longitudinal study of bed sharing and sleep problems among Swiss children in the first 10 years of life. Pediatrics 2005;115:233–40.

Johns MW. A new method for measuring daytime sleepiness: The Epworth sleepiness scale. Sleep 1991;14:541–45.

Johnson JG, Cohen P, Kasen S, First MB, Brook JS. Association between television viewing and sleep problems during adolescence and early adulthood. Arch Pediatr Adolesc Med 2004;158:562–68.

Kahn A, Dan B, Groswasser J, et al. Normal sleep architecture in infants and children. Journal of Clinical Neurophysiology 1996;13(3):184–97.

Kennedy JD, Waters KA. Investigation and treatment of upper-airway obstruction: childhood sleep disorders, part I. Medical Journal of Australia 2005;182(8):419–22.

Kohyama J, Matsukura F, Kimura K, Tachibana N. Rhythmic movement disorder: Polysomnographic study and summary of reported cases. Brain & Development 2002;24:33–38.

Kotagel S, Pianosi P. Sleep disorders in children and adolescents. BMJ 2006;332:828–32.

Kotagal S, Silber MH, Childhood-onset restless legs syndrome. Ann Neurol 2004;56:803–07.

Kristensen G, Jensen IN. Meta-analyses of results of alarm treatment for nocturnal enuresis. Scand J Urol Nephrol 2003;37:232–38.

Kuhn BR, Elliot AJ. Treatment efficacy in behavioral pediatric sleep medicine. Journal of Psychosomatic Resaerch 2003;54:587–97.

Laberge L, Tremblay RE, Vitaro F, Montplaisir J. Development of parasomnias from childhood to early adolescence. Pediatrics 2000;106(1):67–74.

Leduc D and community paediatrics committee. Recommendations for safe sleeping environments for infants and children. Paediatric Child Health 2004;9(9):659–63.

Lee K, Zaffke ME, McEnany G. Parity and sleep patterns during and after pregnancy. Obstetr. Gynecol 2000;95:14–18.

Lipton AJ, Gozal D. Treatment of obstructive sleep apnea in children: Do we really know how? Sleep Med Rev 2003;7(1):61–80.

Lozoff B, Zuckerman B. Sleep problems in children. Pediatrics in Review 1988;10(1):17–24.

Lucassen PLBJ, Assendelft WJJ, Gubbels JW, van Eijk JTM, va Geldrop WJ, Knuistingh Neven A. Effectiveness of treatments for infantile colic: A systemic review. BMJ 1998;316:1563–69.

Mahowald MW, Schenck CH. Parasomnias including the restless legs syndrome. Clinics in Chest Medicine 1998;19(1):183–202.

Mao A, Burnham MM, Goodlin-Jones BL, Gaylor EE, Anders TF. A comparison of the sleep-wake patterns of cosleeping and solitary-sleeping infants. Child Psychiatry & Human Development 2004;35(2):95–105.

Marcus CL, Chapman D, Ward SD, McColey SA, et al. Clinical practice guideline: Diagnosis and management of childhood obstructive sleep apnea syndrome. Pediatrics 2002;109(4):704–12.

Marcus CL. Sleep-disordered breathing in children. Am. J.Respir. Crit. Care Medicine 2001;164:16–30.

Martinez S, Guilleminault C. Periodic leg movements in prepubertal children with sleep disturbance. Developmental Medicine & Child Neurology 2004;46:765–70.

McKay, P. 100 Ways to Calm the Crying. Australia: Griffin Press, 2002.

Mckenna JJ, McDade T. Why babies should never sleep alone: A review of the co-sleeping controversy on relation to SIDS, bedsharing and breast feeding. Paediatric Respiratory Reviews 2005;6:134–52.

Meltzer LJ, Mindell JA. Nonpharmacologic treatments for pediatric sleeplessness. The Pediatric Clinics of North America 2004;51;1:135–52.

Mignot E. A year in review: Basic science, narcolepsy, and sleep in neurologic diseases. Sleep 2004;27(6):1209–12.

Millman RP. Excessive sleepiness in adolescents and young adults: causes, consequences and treatment strategies. Pediatrics 2005;115(6):1774–86.

Mindell JA, Barrett KM. Nightmares and anxiety in elementary-aged children: is there a relationship? Child: Care, Health & Development 2002;28(4):317–22.

Mindell JA, Jacobson BJ. Sleep disturbances during pregnancy. J. Obstet Gynecol Neonatal Nurs 2000;29:590–97.

Mindell JA, Owens JA. A Clinical Guide to Pediatric Sleep. Philadelphia, PA: Lippincott Williams & Wilkins, 2003.

Mirmiran M, Mass YGH, Ariagno RL. Development of fetal and neonatal sleep and circadian rhythms. Sleep Medi Rev 2003;7(4):321–34.

Molin ML, Broch L, Zak R, Gross V. Sleep in women across the life cycle from adulthood through menopause. Sleep Medi Rev 2003;7(2):155–77.

Morin CM, Culbert JP, Schwartz SM. Nonpharmacological interventions for insomnia: A meta-analysis of treatment efficacy. Am J Psychiatry 1994;151:1172–80.

Morin CM, Hauri PJ, Espie CA Spielman A, Duysse DJ, Bootzin R. Nonpharmacologic treatment of chronic insomnia. Sleep 1999;22(8):1–13.

Muris P, Merckelbach, Ollendick TH, King NJ, Bogie N. Children's nighttime fears: Parent-child ratings of frequency, content, origins, coping behaviors and severity. Behavior Research and Therapy 2001;39:13–28.

Odin P. Mrowka M, Shing M. Restless legs syndrome. European Jn. of Neurology 2002;9(3):59–67.

Ohayon MM, Guilleminault C, Preist RG. Night terrors, sleepwalking, and confusional arousals in the general population: Their frequency and relationship to other sleep and mental disorders. J Clin Psychiatry 1999;60:268–76.

Ohayon MM, et al. Meta-analysis of quantitative sleep parameters from childhood to old age in healthy individuals: Developing normative sleep values across the human lifespan. Sleep 2004;27(7):1255–73.

Okawa M, Uchiyama M, Ozaki S et al. Circadian rhythm sleep disorders in adolescents: Clinical trials of combined treatments based on chronobiology. Psychiatry and Clinical Neurosciences 1998;52:483–490.

Owens JA, Babcock D, Blumer J, Chervin R, Ferber R, Goetting M et al. The use of pharmacotherapy in the treatment of pediatrics insomnia in primary care: Rational approaches. A consensus meeting summary. Journal of Clinical Sleep Medicine 2005;1(1):49–59.

Owens JA. Introduction: Culture and sleep in children. Pediatrics 2005;115(1):201–03.

Owens JL, France KG, Wiggs L. Behavioral and cognitive-behavioral interventions for sleep disorders in infants and children: A review. Sleep Medicine Reviews 1999;3(4):281–302.

Pandolfini C, Bonati M, A literature review on off-label drug use in children. Eur J Pediatr 2005;164:552–58.

Pelayo R, Chen W, Monzon S, Guilleminault C. Pediatric sleep pharmacology: You want to give my kid sleeping pills? The Pediatric Clinics of North America 2004;51(1):117–34.

Picchietti DL, Walters AS. Moderate to severe periodic sleep movement disorder in childhood and adolescence. Sleep 1999;22(3):297–300.

Picchietti DL, Underwood DJ, Farris WA, et al. Further studies on periodic limb movement disorder and restless legs syndrome in children with attention-deficit hyperactivity disorder. Movement Disorders 1999;14(6):1000–07.

Ponti M, and Community Pediatrics Committee. Recommendations for the use of pacifiers. Paediatrics & Child Health 2003;8(8):515–19.

Primhak R, O'Brien C. Sleep Apnoea. Arch Dis Child Educ Pract Ed 2005;90:ep87–91.

Reid KJ, Chang AM, Zee PC, et al. Circadian rhythm sleep disorders. Med Clin Am 2004;88:631–51.

Rivkees SA, Mechanisms and clinical significance of circadian rhythms in children. Current Opin Pediatr 2001;13:352–57.

Rosen CL. Obstructive sleep apnea syndrome in children: Controversies in diagnosis and treatment. The Pediatric Clinics of North America 2004;51(1):153–68.

Sadeh A. Assessment of intervention for infant night walking: Parental reports and activity-based home monitoring. Journal of Consulting and Clinical Psychology 1994;62(1):63–68.

Sadeh A. Cognitive-behavioral treatment for childhood sleep disorders. Clinical Psychology Review 2005;25:612–28.

Santiago JR, Nolledo MS, Kinzler W, Santiago T. Sleep and sleep disorders during pregnancy. An Intern Med 2001;134:396–408.

Scheers NJ, Rutheford GS, Kemp JS. Where should infants sleep? A comparision of risk for suffocation of infants sleeping in cribs, adult beds, and other sleeping locations. Pediatrics 2003;112:883–89.

Scher A. Infant sleep at 10 months of age as a window to cognitive development. Early Human Development 2005;81:289–92.

Scher A, Tirosh E, Lavie P. The relationship between sleep and temperament revisited: Evidence for 12 mos olds: A research note. J Child Psychol Psychiat 1998;39(5):785–88.

Sharma V, Mazmanian D. Sleep loss and postpartum psychosis. Bipolar Disorders 2003;5(2):98–105.

Silber MH. Chronic insomnia. NEJM 2005;353:803–10.

Smedje H, Broman J, Hette J. Parents' reports of disturbed sleep in 5-7-year-old Swedish children. Acta Paediatr 1999;88:858–65.

Spruyt K, O'Brien LM, Cluydts R, Verleye GB, Ferri R. Odds, prevalence and predictors of sleep problems in school-age normal children. J. Sleep Res. 2005;14:163–76.

Stein MA, Mandelsohn J, Obermeyer WH et al. Sleep and behavior problems in school-age children. Pediatrics 2001;107(4):E 60

Symon BG, Marley JE, Martin AJ et al. Effect of a consultation teaching behaviour modifications on sleep performance in infants: a randomized controlled trial. MJA 2005; 182(5):215–18.

Tal A, Bar A, Leiberman A, et al. Sleep characteristics following adenotonsillectomy in children with obstructive sleep apnea syndrome. Chest 2003;124:948–53.

Tappin D, Ecob R, Stat S, Brooke H . Bedsharing, roomsharing, and sudden infant death syndrome in Scotland: A case-control study. J Pediatr 2005;147:32–37.

Taras H, Potts-Dema W. Sleep and student performance at school. J. School Health 2005;75(7):248–54.

Task Force on Sudden Infant Death Syndrome. The changing concept of sudden infant death syndrome: Diagnostic coding shifts, controversies regarding the sleeping environment and new variable to consider in reducing risks. Pediatrics 2005;116:1245–55.

Thomas KA, Foreman SW. Infant sleep and feeding pattern: Effects on maternal sleep. J Midwifery Women's Health 2005;50:399–404.

Thome M, Skuladottir A. Evaluating a family-centered intervention for infant sleep problems. Journal of Advanced Nursing 2005;50(1):5–11.

Traeger N, Schultz B, Pollock AN, Mason T, Marcus CL, Arens R. Polysomnographic values in children 2-9 years old: Additional data and review of the literature. Ped Pulmonology 2005;40:22–30.

Trenkwalder C, Paulus W, Walters AS. The restless legs syndrome. The Lancet. Neurology 2005;4:465–75.

U.S. Xyrem Multicenter Study Group. Sodium oxybate demonstrates long-term efficacy for the treatment of cataplexy in patients with narcolepsy. Sleep Medicine 2004;5:119–23.

Walters AS, Mandelbaum DE, Lewin DS, Kugler S, England SJ, Miller M and the Dopaminergic Therapy Study Group. Dopaminergic therapy in children with restless legs/periodic limb movements in sleep and ADHD. Pediatric Neurology 2000;22(3):182–86.

Walters AS. Is there a subpopulation of children with growing pains who really have restless legs syndrome? A review of the literature. Sleep Medicine 2002;3:92–98.

Willinger M, James LS, Catz C. Defining the sudden infant death syndrome (SIDS): deliberations of an expert panel convened by the National Institute of Child Health and Human Development. Pediatr Pathol 1991;11:677–84

Wise MS, Lynch J. Narcolepsy in children. Seminars in Pediatric Neurology 2001;8(4):198–206.

Wolfson AR Carskadon MA. Sleep schedules and daytime functioning in adolescents. Child Development 1998;69(4):875–87.

Wolfson AR, Carskadon MA. Understanding adolescents' sleep patterns and school performance: a critical appraisal. Sleep Medicine Reviews 2003;7(6):491–506.

Wyatt J. Delayed sleep phase syndrome: Pathophysiology and treatment options. Sleep 2004;27(6):1195–203.

Zai C, Wigg KG, Barr CL, Genetics and sleep disorders. Seminars in Clinical Neuropsychiatry 2000;5(1):33–43.

Zeman A, Britton T, Douglas N, Hansen A, Hicks J, Howard R, et.al. Narcolepsy and excessive daytime sleepiness. BMJ 2005;329:724–28.

Acknowledgments

There are many people to acknowledge and thank for their contribution to this book, including:

My colleagues and co-authors who wrote excellent chapters based on their clinical and research expertise, as well as their careful review of the current literature in pediatric sleep medicine.

My colleagues who reviewed chapters and provided valuable insight and thoughtful comments: Drs. Morton Goldbach, Gilles Lavigne, James MacFarlane, Golda Milo-Manson, Janet Nykaza, Evangeline Wassmer, and especially Dr. Robyn Stremler.

Drs. Hugh O'Brodovich and Carter Snead, who supported this project. Other colleagues at The Hospital for Sick Children (HSC), including the sleep technologists and administrative staff of the HSC Sleep Clinic and HSC Sleep Laboratory, who dedicate themselves tirelessly to the patients and families that we care for, as well as Ms. Laura Toth, who provided administrative support.

Dr. Harvey Moldofsky, who has been my mentor in sleep medicine.

The families and children who put their trust in us, not only allowing us to teach them about sleep in children, but also becoming our teachers.

Finally, on behalf of myself and my co-authors, we are grateful for the support and guidance of our publisher, Bob Dees at Robert Rose Inc., Bob Hilderley, senior editor, and Fina Scroppo, copyeditor, as well as the design team at PageWave Graphics. We gratefully acknowledge our editors for their patience, insight, creativity, and thoughtful suggestions, allowing us to present this book in a format that provides our readers with knowledge and strategies to improve the sleep of their children and families.

Index

A

acid reflux (heartburn), 150, 151, 184–85
activities
  before bed, 40, 41, 175
  social, 17
adenoids, 180, 181, 186, 187–88
ADHD (attention deficit/hyperactivity
    disorder), 205
adolescents, 54
  and bed-wetting, 194–95
  inadequate sleep in, 32–33, 228
  insomnia in, 226, 229–34
  nighttime fears of, 173
  sleep disorders of, 76–77, 142
  sleep patterns of, 25–26, 43, 134
  sleepiness in, 226–34
advanced sleep phase syndrome, 73, 140–41,
    147
alcohol, 46, 77
allergies, 151, 209
antihistamines, 84, 203
anxiety, 74, 76, 122, 168, 209. *See also*
    nightmares; nighttime fears
  and panic attacks, 177, 205
apnea, sleep, 184–89. *See also* obstructive
    sleep apnea syndrome
  central, 184–85, 186
  mixed pattern, 184, 186
  treatment guidelines, 186–89
arousal disorders, confusional, 158–67. *See
    also* night terrors; sleepwalking
associations, 106–7, 116–17, 171
  correct, 107–8
  incorrect, 108, 112–14, 117
  parental, 117–23
attention seeking, 214, 216
automatic behavior, 220

B

babies. *See* infants; newborns

bed-sharing, 57–58, 59, 60
  and SIDS, 58, 59
bed-wetting (enuresis), 76, 192–98
  alarm systems for, 86, 194–95
  treatment guidelines, 194–96
bedding, 58, 196
bedroom. *See also* sleep hygiene
  environment of, 41–42, 73, 146, 174
  sharing, 55, 57, 60, 123, 177
bedtime
  activities before, 40, 41, 175
  faded, 79
  routines for, 42–43, 46–54, 97, 116, 143,
    174
behavioral problems, 109, 174
behavioral strategies, 37–40, 51, 78–79, 240.
    See also extinction method
  for bed-wetting, 195–96
  chair-sitting, 118, 121
  during pregnancy, 240
  for teenage sleepiness, 231–33
  timed-waiting, 118–20, 121–22
biofeedback, 233
biological clock, 16–18, 21, 133
  resetting, 143–46, 147
bladder training, 196
bottle-feeding, 101–3
brain, 12, 13, 20–21
  and breathing, 179, 190
breast-feeding, 57, 62, 91, 97–100
breathing, 179, 190
  and oxygen levels, 181, 183
  sleep problems with, 178–91
bright-light therapy, 86
bruxism (teeth grinding/gnashing), 208–12

C

caffeine, 43–44, 203, 204, 207
carrying. *See* holding
cataplexy, 219, 220, 222–23, 225
chair-sitting strategy, 118, 121

children. *See specific age groups*
circadian process (process C), 11, 16–18, 20, 48
circadian rhythms, 133. *See also* sleep phases
co-sleeping, 56–60, 63–65
cognitive behavioral therapy, 240
colic, 150–54
coping skills, 176
corticosteroids, 187
CPAP (continuous positive airway pressure), 189, 239
crying (excessive), 149–57. *See also* colic
    causes, 149–50, 152
    treatment guidelines, 156

D

delayed sleep phase syndrome, 73, 122, 138–46
    symptoms, 138–40
    treatments, 84, 86, 141–46
depression, 77, 235, 238
desmopressin (DDAVP), 195
development, 20–21
    delayed, 213, 215
diaries
    apnea, 181–82
    crying, 152
    sleep, 80–81, 143, 147
diet, 43, 154, 206. *See also* bottle-feeding; breast-feeding; caffeine; overweight; snacks
dopamine, 201, 203
dreaming. *See* REM sleep
drugs. *See also* medications
    illicit, 77
dyssomnias, 68, 70

E

education strategies, 78, 80, 142, 205
emotional problems, 196
energy drinks, 204. *See also* caffeine
enuresis. *See* bed-wetting
environment
    in bedroom, 41–42, 73, 146, 174
    temperature of, 18, 42, 59
Epworth Sleepiness Scale, 227
exercise, 44, 146, 206, 240
extinction ('cold turkey') method, 79, 115
    consistency in, 121, 122
    graduated, 116, 117–23

F

family, 69, 109, 122, 130. *See also* parents
fatigue, 32, 227. *See also* tiredness
fears. *See* anxiety; night terrors; nightmares; nighttime fears
fetus, 18–20, 237, 238

G

growing pains, 207
growth, 12

H

hallucinations, 219
head-banging. *See* rhythmic movement disorder (RMD)
health problems, 68, 77, 84, 109, 123
    and hypoventilation, 190, 191
    neurological, 70, 208
    and sleep disorders, 150, 203, 215
heartburn (acid reflux), 150, 151, 184–85
holding, 151, 153
hormones, 133. *See also* melatonin
hunger, 149
hypnogram, sleep, 15
hypoventilation, 178, 190–91

I

illness, 77, 123. *See also* health problems
imagery (visualization), 233
imipramine, 195
infants (3–12 months)
    co-sleeping with, 56–60
    feeding patterns of, 50–51, 92, 111
    older (6–12 months), 50–52, 72–73
    responding to, 115, 151, 153
    separation anxiety in, 73, 122, 173, 175
    sleep disorders of, 72–73, 111–15
    sleep hygiene for, 48–52, 112
    sleep patterns of, 22–23
    sleeping alone, 113, 114–15
    sleeping position, 59, 60
    younger (4–6 months), 48–49
insomnia
    adolescent, 54, 77, 226, 229–34
    causes, 54, 88–90
    childhood, 88–93
    during pregnancy, 238, 239–40

primary, 77, 229–30
treatment guidelines, 91–92, 231–34
iron deficiency, 203, 206

K
kicking, 204–5

L
light
cycles of, 17, 41
sunlight, 43, 146
therapy using, 86
limit-setting, 129–30, 131, 147
limit-setting disorder, 71, 74, 76, 89, 125–31
causes, 126–28
treatment guidelines, 128–30

M
meal timing, 17, 97–103, 111
medications, 82–86
for apnea, 187
for arousal disorders, 165
for bed-wetting, 195
for insomnia, 233
for narcolepsy, 224
as nightmare cause, 169
over-the-counter, 82, 83, 84, 85
and RLS, 203, 206, 211
melatonin, 84–86, 133
morningness *vs.* eveningness, 136–37
motivational strategies, 142–43
movies, 171
muscles, 190, 205
music
as sleep aid, 40, 153, 232
as sleep disrupter, 41, 89, 108, 115, 146, 231

N
naps, 44, 53, 146. *See also* narcolepsy
infants and, 112, 115
during pregnancy, 239
toddlers and, 23, 24
narcolepsy, 77, 218–25
treatment guidelines, 223–24
neurological disorders, 70, 208. *See also* narcolepsy

newborns (0–3 months)
and circadian process, 11, 20, 48
nurturing, 47, 151, 153
sleep hygiene for, 46–48
sleep patterns of, 11, 20, 48
sleeping position, 59, 60
nicotine, 46, 77. *See also* smoke, secondhand
night terrors, 75, 76, 159–61
nightmares, 74, 76, 168–72
nighttime fears, 74, 76, 173–77
nocturnal eating (drinking) syndrome, 73, 74, 88–89, 93, 94–105
symptoms, 95–96
treatment guidelines, 97–104
noise, 18, 41
NREM (non-rapid eye movement) sleep, 12, 13, 14–16, 27–28

O
obesity. *See* overweight
object permanence, 114, 126
obstructive sleep apnea syndrome (OSAS), 75, 76, 164, 178, 185–86
diary of, 181–82
effects, 186, 237
during pregnancy, 237
surgery for, 86, 187–88
treatment guidelines, 187–89, 239
overtiredness, 149, 153, 156
overweight, 186, 187, 190, 191
oxygen levels, 181, 183

P
pacifiers, 61–63, 108
and SIDS, 61–62
pain, 73, 209, 211
panic attacks, 177, 205
parasomnias, 68, 70
partial arousal, 158–67
treatment guidelines, 163–65
parents
associations with, 117–23
bed-sharing with, 57–58
and bed-wetting, 196
and colic, 150, 154
and limit-setting disorder, 126
room-sharing with, 55, 57
periodic limb movement disorder (PLMD), 199, 200, 205

pets, 177
plagiocephaly, positional, 60
polysomnography. *See* sleep, studies of
postpartum depression, 235
pregnancy, 19–20, 235–41
preschoolers (3–5 years), 24, 52–53, 74, 173
process C. *See* circadian process
process S, 16
psychiatric disorders, 70
punishment. *See* rewards
puzzles, 206

R

reinforcement, positive, 79, 130. *See also*
     rewards
relaxation techniques, 165, 206, 211, 233,
     240
REM (dreaming) sleep, 12–13, 14–16, 25, 27,
     168–69, 219
restless legs syndrome (RLS), 76, 77, 164,
     199–207
   causes, 203
   diagnosis, 200–202
   during pregnancy, 237–38
   treatment for, 84, 205–6, 239
restlessness, 204–5
rewards, 37, 130, 147, 176, 195. *See also*
     reinforcement, positive
rhythmic movement disorder (RMD), 74,
     213–17
RLS. *See* restless legs syndrome
rocking. *See* rhythmic movement disorder
room-sharing, 55, 57, 60, 123, 177
roughhousing, 40, 175
routines
   bedtime, 42–43, 46–54, 97, 116, 143, 174
   and crying, 153, 156

S

safety, 51, 55–65, 154, 177
   guidelines for, 59–60
   sleep disorders and, 164, 165, 216
school-age children (6–12 years), 25, 53,
     75–76, 173
security objects, 171
seizures, 185, 205, 212, 217
self-soothing, 155
self-stimulation, 214
separation anxiety, 73, 122, 173, 175

SIDS (sudden infant death syndrome), 55–56,
     60
   bed-sharing and, 58, 59
   pacifiers and, 61–62
sleep, 10–28. *See also* sleep disorders; sleep
     patterns; sleep phases
   adequate, 30, 31–33, 36–46, 167
   alone, 92, 113, 114–15
   arousals from, 159, 161, 162, 164
   changes during, 12–13
   cycles of, 16–18
   deep (slow-wave), 27, 159, 162, 193
   disturbed, 26, 34, 68, 77, 214, 228–29
   duration, 29, 31–32
   fragmented, 162, 164
   functions, 10–11
   habits of, 37–40, 41–46, 51
   inadequate, 31–35, 164, 171
   need for, 19, 29–35
   during pregnancy, 235–36
   questions about, 26–28
   states of, 12–16
   studies of, 181, 182–83, 200, 224, 225
sleep diaries, 80–81, 143, 147
sleep disorders, 34–35, 69, 70–71
   of adolescents, 76–77, 142
   of children, 73–75, 109–10, 116–23
   consequences, 72
   health problems and, 150, 203, 215
   of infants, 72–73, 111–15
   during pregnancy, 236–41
   and safety, 164, 165, 216
   symptoms, 68–77
   treatments, 78–86
   types, 68, 70
sleep hygiene, 36–54
   improving, 143, 154, 163, 206, 239
   for infants, 48–52, 112
   for newborns, 46–48
   poor-quality, 73, 74, 76
   worksheet on, 39–40
sleep myoclonus, 204–5
sleep-onset association disorder, 73–74, 76,
     89, 93, 106–24
   features, 106–10
   in infants, 111–15
   in toddlers, 109–10, 116–23
   treatment guidelines, 111–15
sleep paralysis, 220
sleep patterns, 18–26, 27–28
   of children, 23–24

cultural context of, 30, 70–71
fetal, 18–20
of infants, 22–23
irregular, 26, 74, 76
of newborns, 11, 20, 48
during pregnancy, 235–36
of teenagers, 25–26, 43, 134
sleep phases, 134–37. *See also* advanced sleep
   phase syndrome; delayed sleep phase
   syndrome
   disorders of, 73–75, 89–90, 132–48
   preferences for, 130, 134, 136–37, 148
sleep restriction therapy, 232–33
sleepiness, 68, 226–34
sleeping pills, 233. *See also* medications
sleeplessness. *See* insomnia
sleepovers, 165, 195
sleepwalking, 75, 161–62, 164, 165
smoke, secondhand, 58, 60, 154, 187
snacks, 43, 45, 174
snoring, 178
special needs. *See* health problems
steroids. *See* corticosteroids
stimulation, 152, 156, 175, 214, 215
stimulus control therapy, 231–32
stress, 84, 123, 209
   reducing, 164, 165, 211
sunlight, 43, 146
surgery, 86, 187–88

T

teenagers. *See* adolescents
teeth grinding/gnashing (bruxism), 208–12
teething, 52, 73
television, 41, 42, 108, 134, 169, 228
temperament, 150, 155–56
temperature, 18, 42, 59, 133
thought stopping, 233
timed-waiting strategy, 118–20, 121–22
tiredness, 149, 153, 156. *See also* fatigue
toddlers (1–3 years), 23–24, 52–53
   co-sleeping with, 63–65
   sleep disorders of, 73–75, 109–10, 116–23
tonsils, 180, 186, 187–88
tracheostomy, 188
training pants, 196
transitional objects, 114
traveling, 123, 165

V

video games, 171, 206

W

waking, 43, 47, 48, 50, 109
weaning, 92, 103–5, 111

Z

zeitgebers, 16–18, 43